Treatment of Hand Injuries

Treatment of Hand Injuries

Preservation and Restoration of Function

Elden C. Weckesser, M.D.

Clinical Professor of Surgery
School of Medicine
Case Western Reserve University

The Press of Case Western Reserve University

Distributed by Year Book Medical Publishers, Inc.
35 East Wacker Drive
Chicago, Illinois 60601

To my wife Kathryn for her help, patience, and understanding, and to my daughters, Jane, Elizabeth, Nancy, and Mary.

Contents

Foreword

The hand, with its infinite capability to bring humans through industrial, professional, and artistic careers, is, like laughter, one of the very few possessions that characterizes man. We all recognize the tragedy experienced by a manual laborer or a concert pianist when he loses the use of a hand. It is hardly less of a catastrophe when disease or trauma disables the hand of an individual who is not dependent upon the exquisite sensory and motor function of his hands in order to earn a living. The thousands of manual and digital exercises of the hand needed to carry out the ordinary and frequently subconscious acts of daily life are only fully appreciated when they are encumbered or lost by disability. To lose unilateral vision or hearing, one kidney, or one lower extremity is unpleasant to say the least, but it is no handicap to living a full and productive life. To lose the function of one hand can be disastrous.

This thoroughly illustrated book by Dr. Weckesser is designed to acquaint physicians who do not daily manage the complexities of trauma and disease of the hand with the basic principles of surgery of the hand. It is suffused with practical recommendations for management that can minimize manual defects and permit a maximal recovery of function. It is based upon an experience of over thirty years wherein the simplest and the most complex of hand problems have both received professional attention and care of the highest quality. The potential this book has for minimizing hand disability is inestimable.

William D. Holden, M.D.
Oliver H. Payne Professor of Surgery
School of Medicine
Case Western Reserve University

Acknowledgments

Appreciation is expressed to: the Donald and Alice Burdett Surgical Fund, the Newbell Niles Puckett Fund, and The Stone Foundation (formerly of Cleveland and now of New York City) for financial support in the preparation of this work; Mrs. Lydia Holian and all members of the staff of the Allen Memorial Medical Library; all the nurses in surgery, without whose help the surgeon's work could not be done, especially Miss Marilyn Yanick and Mrs. June Lorig; Miss Marita Bitans and Mrs. Barbara Rankin for the drawings; my predecessors and contemporaries whose ideas I have been privileged to share; and the staff of the Press of Case Western Reserve University for their invaluable help.

Treatment of Hand Injuries

Introduction

This treatise on the preservation and restoration of function of the hand following injury is intended for the beginning student, the house officer in the early part of his training, and the practitioner who does not treat hand injuries often and, consequently, has not had great experience with them. It offers a ready outline of basic principles. It is intended to provide a proper basis for treatment during the very early stages following injury so that the highest degree of function can be retained and restored. The first treatment and proper immediate aftercare, the immediate referral when this is essential, and the pitfalls to avoid are indicated. It is also intended to offer a sound basis on which to build a detailed interest and knowledge of surgery of the hand for the student who wishes to go further into this field.

The preservation and restoration of function of the hand—the exquisite sense of touch and strong but refined movement—is the goal for treatment of injuries to this part of the body. The hand is an organ of action. It must be able to do things. Physical restoration of its parts is not enough. The parts must be restored in such a way that they work. Without detracting from the importance of anatomy and the anatomical charts which follow, emphasis throughout this book is placed upon function. The two essential functions of the hand readily lost by injury are:

1. Mobility
2. Sensitivity

The concentration of bones distally in the upper extremity (figure 1) allows unique mobility. Of the thirty or more bones involved, all but the three largest ones are located in or distal to the wrist. The many small joints between these bones have been highly developed in the upper extremity for the movements of grasp and manipulation. The movement of these small joints essential for full hand function and movement, allowed by small collateral ligaments and elastic joint capsules, is readily lost by injury or immobilization. The fifteen joints of the fingers and thumb each have small clearance in their joint spaces. Small amounts of shortening in their collateral ligaments and capsules—the result of injury or immobilization—interfere more with movement than similar changes in larger joints. In addition to this, the four fingers act as a team for many of their functions, and a limitation of movement in one interferes with the function of the other. Joint mobility, tendon gliding, and muscle contractility are all highly essential functions which deserve every surgical effort to preserve and restore.

Pain sensation protects, and the acute touch sensation of the fingertips gives information about the texture and shape of things which cannot be obtained in any other way. It allows the hand to

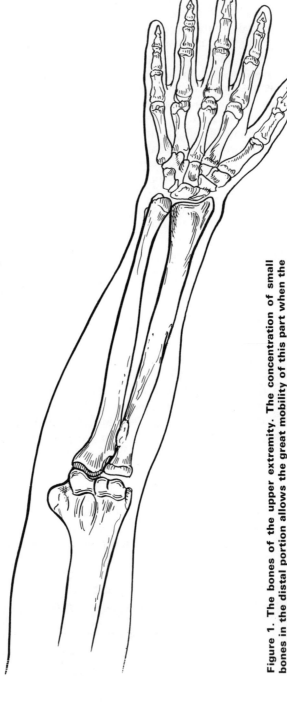

Figure 1. The bones of the upper extremity. The concentration of small bones in the distal portion allows the great mobility of this part when the fine joints between them are supple and supplied by normal nerve muscle tendon motor units. All but three bones are distal to the wrist.

function even in complete darkness and, more important, allows the hand to function without direct vision, freeing the eyes for other simultaneous uses.

While the title of this book refers only to treatment of hand injuries, the book actually deals with the treatment of patients with injuries of the hand. The physician's awareness of the entire patient is essential. Injuries to other parts of the body, constitutional disease, and the patient's psychological reactions must all be considered in each case, especially if the injury is severe. The hand and the brain are closely interrelated, and severe psychological reaction to severe injury is frequent. Any person dependent upon the skills of his hands for his livelihood may be thrown into extreme depression by such an injury.

Because it is an active and essential part of so much of what we do, the upper extremity and especially the hands are in jeopardy more than many other parts of the body. The marvels of mechanized society bring many additional hazards to man, and no small part of these are injuries to the upper extremity. According to *Accident Facts*, published by the National Safety Council, nearly one-third of all "lost time" industrial injuries involve the upper extremity. This is greater even than the percentage of injuries to the trunk of the body.

Mechanization has also made the types of injury more severe. Power tools are more destructive than hand tools. In recent years, I have seen increasing numbers of severe mangling injuries of the upper extremity. This does not mean that safety measures cannot be, or are not, effective in the prevention of accidents. Available data indicate very definitely that safety measures are effective and, hence, that they should be stressed in industry to offset the trend toward greater numbers of, and more extensive, injuries.

Of the injuries to the hand, injuries to skin and subcutaneous tissue are most frequent. These carry dirt, grease, foreign bodies, and "all sorts of things" deep beneath the skin where infection is very prone to develop. Infections in the hand are a serious hazard to hand function. They can be almost completely avoided by immediate cleansing, irrigation with normal saline solution, debridement, primary closure, and judicious antibiotics, as described in chapter 1.

The next most frequent injury about the hand is tendon laceration, because the tendons are taut and, for this reason, divided more readily by sharp objects. Loss of tendon action means loss of movement and loss of function. These injuries require the same early cleansing, wound irrigation, debridement, and search for foreign bodies, as noted before, to prevent infection. If factors are favorable, early repair can then be carried out (see chapter 8). However, the situation here is complicated by the tendency for lateral adhesions to form, especially in the flexor tunnels of the fingers, which limit function. How to avoid this complication taxes the efforts of even the most experienced. The beginner is advised to refer this problem to the experienced operator.

Nerves are lacerated in nearly half of all tendon injuries. Early or late repair is still controversial, but the tendency in recent years has been toward "immediate" or early repair in clean cases seen by the experienced operator. The problem is to get the regenerating neurons to cross the site of repair before fibroblasts create scar.

Fractures in the hand require accurate reduction, perhaps more so than in some other parts of the body, since the clearance of the many small finger and thumb joints is small. Open reduction is

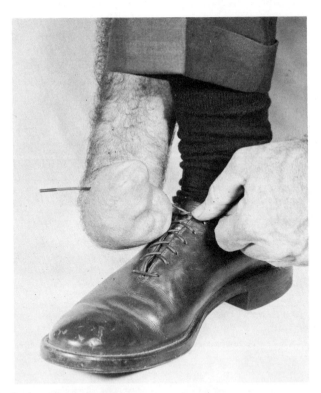

Figure 2. Forty-three-year-old man whose right hand had been amputated, at age seven, in a silage cutter. The wrist joint and one metacarpal remained. He developed grasp by flexing the remaining metacarpal against his forearm, as shown. This is an extreme example of what is possible with mobile sensitive parts when injury occurs in childhood.

usually advocated for this reason and also to allow earlier movement and, thus prevent the spector of joint stiffness which can destroy hand function.

Severe crush injuries, although fortunately less frequent, are destructive of all elements of the hand. The efforts here must be to maintain some elements for grasp which will have sensation. Any remaining functional parts with normal sensation are better than a prosthesis (figure 2).

It is hoped that this compilation, representing knowledge gained over the past thirty years, may help others to diminish the crippling effects of hand injuries. Hand injuries are not a threat to life, but a tremendous threat to livelihood.

ANATOMY OF THE UPPER EXTREMITIES

(These anatomical diagrams are included for review and reference.)

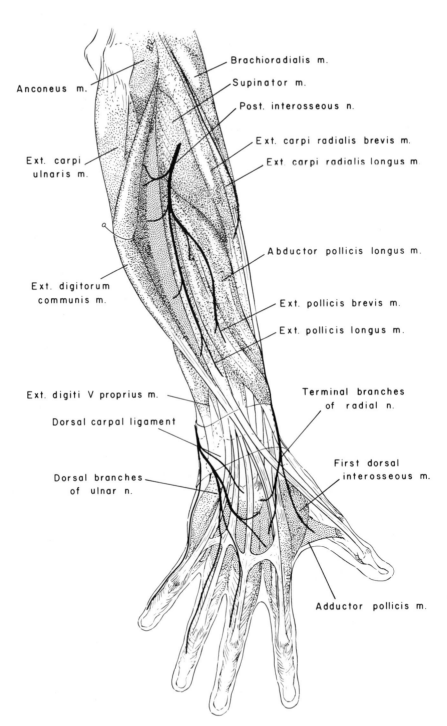

Anconeus m.

Ext. carpi
ulnaris m.

Ext. digitorum
communis m.

Ext. digiti V proprius m.

Dorsal carpal ligament

Dorsal branches
of ulnar n.

Brachioradialis m.

Supinator m.

Post. interosseous n.

Ext. carpi radialis brevis m.

Ext. carpi radialis longus m.

Abductor pollicis longus m.

Ext. pollicis brevis m.

Ext. pollicis longus m.

Terminal branches
of radial n.

First dorsal
interosseous m.

Adductor pollicis m.

Figure 3. Dorsal aspect of forearm and hand. Diagrammatic representation of muscles and tendons.

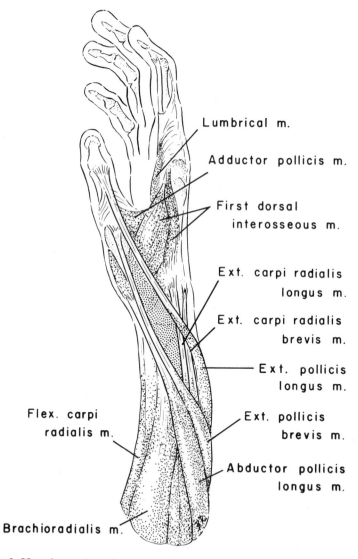

Lumbrical m.

Adductor pollicis m.

First dorsal
interosseous m.

Ext. carpi radialis
longus m.

Ext. carpi radialis
brevis m.

Ext. pollicis
longus m.

Flex. carpi
radialis m.

Ext. pollicis
brevis m.

Abductor pollicis
longus m.

Brachioradialis m.

Figure 4. Muscles and tendons of radial aspect of the wrist.

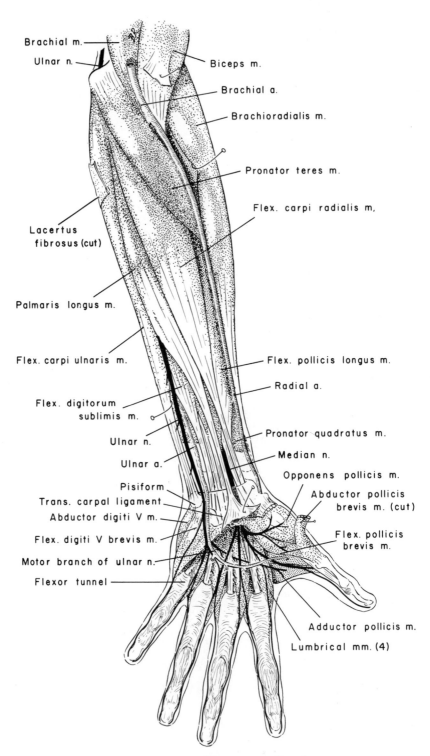

Brachial m.

Ulnar n.

Biceps m.

Brachial a.

Brachioradialis m.

Pronator teres m.

Flex. carpi radialis m.

Lacertus
fibrosus (cut)

Palmaris longus m.

Flex. carpi ulnaris m.

Flex. pollicis longus m.

Radial a.

Flex. digitorum
sublimis m.

Pronator quadratus m.

Ulnar n.

Median n.

Ulnar a.

Opponens pollicis m.

Pisiform

Trans. carpal ligament

Abductor pollicis
brevis m. (cut)

Abductor digiti V m.

Flex. pollicis
brevis m.

Flex. digiti V brevis m.

Motor branch of ulnar n.

Flexor tunnel

Adductor pollicis m.

Lumbrical mm. (4)

Figure 5. Superficial volar aspect of forearm and hand.

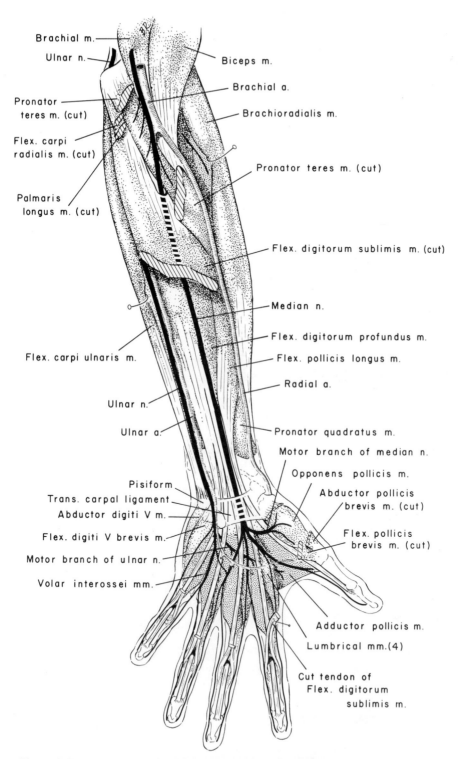

Brachial m.

Ulnar n.

Biceps m.

Brachial a.

Pronator
teres m. (cut)

Brachioradialis m.

Flex. carpi
radialis m. (cut)

Pronator teres m. (cut)

Palmaris
longus m. (cut)

Flex. digitorum sublimis m. (cut)

Median n.

Flex. digitorum profundus m.

Flex. pollicis longus m.

Flex. carpi ulnaris m.

Radial a.

Ulnar n.

Ulnar a.

Pronator quadratus m.

Motor branch of median n.

Opponens pollicis m.

Pisiform

Trans. carpal ligament

Abductor pollicis
brevis m. (cut)

Abductor digiti V m.

Flex. digiti V brevis m.

Flex. pollicis
brevis m. (cut)

Motor branch of ulnar n.

Volar interossei mm.

Adductor pollicis m.

Lumbrical mm.(4)

Cut tendon of
Flex. digitorum
sublimis m.

**Figure 6. Deep volar aspect of forearm and hand. The sublimis muscle bellies
have been removed to show structures beneath them.**

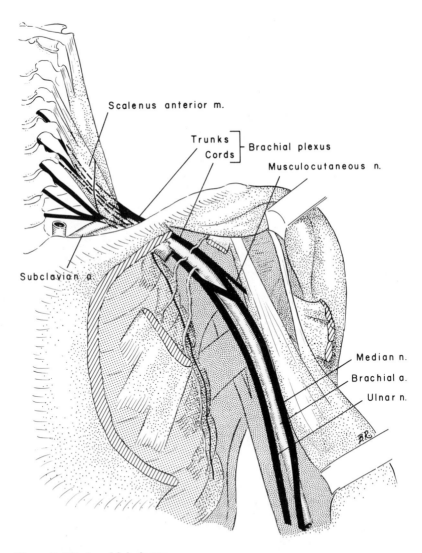

Figure 7. The brachial plexus.

CHAPTER 1

Primary Treatment of the Injured Patient with Wounds of the Upper Extremity, Including Care of the Wound

---

ABSTRACT

The anatomical parts of the hand—small, delicate, and closely packed together—are readily injured. Hemorrhage can be controlled by local pressure or the application of a pneumatic cuff tourniquet above the wound. The use of a pneumatic cuff tourniquet to produce a bloodless field for ninety minutes or less during the surgical repair of traumatic wounds and surgical operations is highly desirable. A head loupe with two-diameter magnification is a great aid in the gentle handling of tissues during cleansing and debridement.

Care of the vital functions of the injured patient—respiration and circulation—are of first importance. An overall evaluation of the patient is next. Determine how, when, and where the wound occurred. Test function distally rather than probe the wound. Check it out as follows:

1. *Test tendon movement of each joint distal to the wound.*
2. *Test sensation distal to wound:*
   pinprick
   Weber 2-point
3. *Test function of intrinsic muscles of the hand:*
   opponens muscle (motor median)
   first dorsal interosseous (motor ulnar)
4. *X ray for fracture when indicated.*

Extensive cleansing under block or general anesthesia should be done in two stages.

Debride with caution, preserving essential parts. Definitive tendon and nerve repair should be done in early clean cases only.

Skin closure only should be done after debridement and cleansing if the case is contaminated, the time-lapse is more than a few hours after injury, or the operator is not familiar with tendon and nerve repair.

In very contaminated cases, bite wounds, or blast wounds, the wound should be left open, and local and systemic antibiotics should be given. Systemic immunization, such as tetanus toxoid, should also be given.

Pitfalls

1. *Infection because of improperly cleansed and irrigated wound*
2. *Overlooked serious damage to tendons and nerves from what appears to be an innocuous cut on the skin*
3. *Overlooked tendon division because of failure to test tendon function distal to the wound*
4. *Overlooked nerve injury because of failure to test pinprick and 2-point sensation distal to the wound (In children, ninhydrin or starch tests may be needed.)*
5. *Overlooked fracture*
6. *Overlooked foreign body*
7. *Avulsed tendon base of distal phalanx:*
    extensor (mallet finger deformity)
    flexor profundus (no deformity, but lack of active flexion of the distal joint)
8. *A long skin flap with narrow base, especially if the base is located distally*
9. *Unrecognized other serious injury in patient*
10. *Unnecessarily immobilized joints, which lead to stiffness*
11. *Delay of treatment for grease- or paint-injection injury*
12. *Severe vascular damage associated with roller injury*

Types of Cases Best Referred to Experienced Operator Early

1. *Divided tendon in No Man's Land*
2. *Extensive injury of skin, tendon, nerve, bone, or joint*
3. *Avulsion of skin of entire digit or digits*
4. *Displaced fracture of proximal phalanx*

The treatment of wounds of the upper extremity, as urgent and demanding as it frequently is, cannot proceed without consideration at the same time for other possible injuries or conditions in the patient. The following is an outline of proper procedure to ensure that priorities are observed and correlated when a patient is first seen:

1. Control of hemorrhage and assurance of respiratory function (associated injuries)

2. Overall evaluation of patient
3. History (how, when, where)
4. Evaluation of extent of injury to extremity
   a. Only minimal examination of wound
   b. Tests for function distal to point of injury:
      tendons
      nerves (sensory and motor)
5. Treatment indicated
   a. Recent injury seen early: to surgery
   b. Remote injury (seen late) with suppuration:
      hospitalization
      heat, rest, elevation, drainage, antibiotics
6. Postoperative care
   a. Specific immunizations
   b. Antibiotics
   c. Elevation

CONTROL OF HEMORRHAGE AND ASSURANCE OF RESPIRATORY FUNCTION

Hemorrhage and respiratory dysfunction are the two real emergencies in in any injured patient and must be attended to first. The quickest method to control hemorrhage is by direct pressure on the wound by sterile gauze or the cleanest material available. The effectiveness of this method is attested every day in the operating room. The dressing may be bandaged firmly in place for a short interval of time, up to one and one-half hours. However, when the patient is brought to the hospital, the readily available pneumatic cuff tourniquet is preferable when inflated to 100 mm Hg above the systolic pressure. It can also be left in place for a similar period of time, which should be more than adequate for definitive treatment to get under way. When large vessels are divided, the ultimate, of course, is repair of the injured vessel under the best circumstances of light, exposure, and magnification. Ligation is resorted to only if the remaining circulation is adequate and the vessel is small and unimportant.

The airway should be cleared and any associated wound of the respiratory tree or thorax so treated to restore respiratory exchange at the earliest possible time.

OVERALL EVALUATION OF THE PATIENT

A danger to the life of the patient exists if the patient's overall condition is overlooked. Overall evaluation need not be time-consuming, but must proceed carefully to determine if a more serious injury exists elsewhere. After overall evaluation of the patient has been made, proper treatment of the upper extremity wound must proceed as an early priority, for infection is greatly inhibited—often avoided—by wound cleansing and early wound closure.

HISTORY

The *how, when,* and *where* of the accident should be elicited and recorded, as each of these factors is important. The mode of injury contributes greatly to the condition of the wound at the time it is seen and may be a decisive factor in choosing the type of treatment. A clean, incised wound made by a sharp blade is far different from a ragged, torn wound produced by a saw or chain or some other blunt instrument. Where the injury occurred is equally important, because the degree of contamination will be directly related to this. A wound that occurs in a street heavily contaminated with all sorts of organisms is far different from a wound that occurs at home in the kitchen or under other clean circumstances. The time of injury is important for different reasons. Organisms begin to multiply immediately after introduction into a wound, and the length of time which has elapsed is thus very important and very relevant to the proper treatment. Dr. Sumner Koch, of Chicago, has spoken of the first four to six hours after injury as the "golden interval" during which time clean wounds can be irrigated and converted to closed wounds with nearly the same hazard of infection as aseptically made wounds. Primary repair of divided structures may be carried out during this early "golden interval" in properly selected cases.

EVALUATION OF EXTENT OF
INJURY TO THE EXTREMITY

In order to determine what structures have been divided, the first impulse of the examiner is to look at the wound itself. This usually does not supply the information that the examiner wishes:
1. Exposure is very poor.
2. Hemorrhage and much blood obscure the structures in the wound.
3. Many structures retract out of sight.

Furthermore, additional damage may be inflicted, and additional contamination may be introduced.

For these reasons, it is wiser to carry out functional tests distal to the wound. These functional tests, as shown in the procedure outline on page 17 should involve the tendons and the nerves in particular. Keep in mind that the profundus tendons primarily flex the distal joints of the fingers. Each finger should be held proximal to the distal joint and the patient then asked to flex this articulation. In cases of injury to the sublimis tendons, which primarily flex the middle joints of the fingers, the proximal interphalangeal (p.i.p.) joints, the situation is not as clear-cut because the profundus tendons also traverse this joint and have

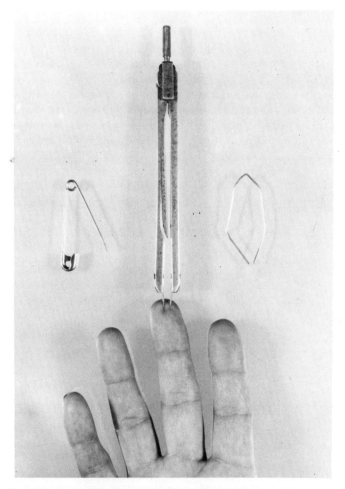

Figure 1–1. Sensory function is tested with the blunt and sharp end of a safety pin, asking the patient to identify each. The two points of a compass or bent paper clip, set at 3–4 mm, are an excellent additional test for nerve function, switching from one to two points and asking the patient, without the help of vision, to identify which it is.

action upon it. But because the profundus tendons usually have a common muscle belly, if the adjacent fingers are held in hyperextension the function of the profundus tendon on the middle finger joint is negated and the flexion of this joint will show that the sublimis tendon is still functioning. This is usually the case; however, some people have independent action of the profundus tendons, especially to the index finger, and in cases such as these the test for sublimis function is not valid.

If the wound is above the wrist, of course the appropriate tendons that move that joint should be tested specifically.

Nerve function should be tested, both sensory and motor (figure 1–1 and figure 1–2). Sensory function is quickly tested with a safety pin; the sharp end and the blunt end can be readily interchanged, and the ability of the patient to distinguish the two, without the help of vision, can be determined (figure 1–1).

The Weber 2-point discrimination test determines the patient's ability to detect the presence of two points 3 to 4 mm apart on the skin surface. It is a very useful test which can be carried out

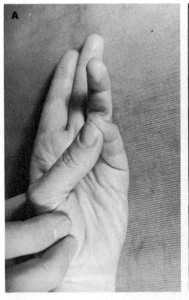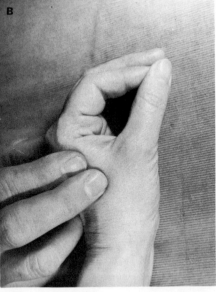

Figure 1–2. Intrinsic muscle tests of the hand. *A*, the motor fibers of the median nerve supplying intrinsic muscles of the hand are readily tested by palpating the contraction of the opponens muscle of the thumb. *B*, the motor fibers of the ulnar nerve are similarly tested by palpating contracture of the first dorsal interosseous muscle which abducts the index finger. Both are objective tests.

with a caliper or a bent paper clip. It is more critical than the pinprick test and is useful in determining minor injuries, but the ability to distinguish two points is lost before point-prick in partial injuries of the sensory nerves.[9]

The occurrence of perspiration on the part being tested has been shown to correspond to an area with intact peripheral nerves. This has been the basis of the print tests with starch-iodine or with ninhydrin. An area which perspires will make a positive fingerprint test with either of these methods. The starch-iodine test depends upon the moisture on the tested fingertip creating a blue color between the starch and the iodine in the test paper. Ninhydrin is a sensitive reagent which makes a dark stain with amino acids and lower peptides. The prints are made on nonporous plain white writing paper and developed with special reagents. The techniques[8] for both of these tests are included here.

TECHNIQUE OF NINHYDRIN FINGERPRINT TEST

1. Make patient perspire using one or more of these methods:
   Give hot tea or coffee
   Place in warm room
   Have patient exercise
   Do pinprick test
2. Print fingertips, one at a time, on a sheet of dry nonporous paper 3 × 15 cm. Outline fingertips with pencil.
3. Develop fingerprint, dip paper in shallow dish containing 1% ninhydrin in acetone solution with a few drops of glacial acetic acid per 10 ml.
4. Dry paper strips and warm to between 100° and 120° for five to ten minutes.
5. Read print.
6. Make fixation, preferably three days later. Dip paper strips in 1% solution copper nitrate in 5:95 mixture of water and methyl alcohol or acetone acidified with a few drops concentrated nitric acid per 100 ml.

TECHNIQUE OF STARCH-IODINE FINGERPRINT TEST

1. Make patient perspire as in the test for ninhydrin.
2. Print fingertips and outline, same special paper impregnated with starch and iodine.
3. Read print immediately.
4. Photograph for record, if desired.

The starch-iodine print can be read immediately and need not be developed.

It sometimes gives more distinct dots for the sweat glands, but lasts only several weeks. The fixed ninhydrin prints are equally valuable to determine nerve function but have the advantage in that they are permanent and can be stored.[8]

Absent pseudomotor function indicates areas of anesthesia. The ninhydrin test requires a number of chemical reagents which may not always be available, but it is certainly a worthwhile test, especially for children. I prefer the pinprick test and looking for visible and palpable perspiration on the fingertips. The Weber 2-point test is most useful during recovery, to determine the extent of regeneration.

Testing for motor function of the intrinsic muscles of the hand is readily carried out. Since the radial nerve supplies no intrinsic muscles in the hand normally, the motor tests of intrinsic musculature are confined to determining injury to the median and ulnar nerves.

Motor Function of the Ulnar Nerve

The ulnar nerve supplies all the interosseous muscles of the hand. The first dorsal interosseous muscle of the radial side of the index finger metacarpal is readily palpable. An objective test of ulnar nerve motor function is to palpate the muscle belly of the first dorsal interosseous muscle while asking the patient to alternately abduct and adduct the index finger. This muscle can be readily palpated as it contracts beneath the fingertips, making this an objective test (figure 1–2). An alternative method is to ask the patient to pinch between the thumb and index finger; the examiner will feel the first dorsal interosseous muscle contract when this function is carried out.

Motor Function of the Median Nerve

Since the median nerve sends a motor branch to the thenar eminence (to the opponens muscle) immediately after passing under the transverse carpal ligament, the motor function of the opponens muscle can be objectively evaluated in a similar manner to the first dorsal interosseous muscle by palpating the opponens muscle as the thumb is brought into opposition. The alternative method of testing the ulnar motor function (as described before) can also be utilized because, on bringing the thumb and the index finger together in pinch, the opponens muscle tightens along with the first dorsal interosseous muscle utilized in this maneuver.

These motor function tests of the intrinsic muscles can be readily carried out in a very short period of time and are very useful in conjunction with the determination of sensation in the digits.

As shown in the procedure outline (page 17), after evaluation of the extent of injury a decision should be made regarding definitive surgery of deep structures. The first consideration before such surgery must be the time-lapse since injury. A recent injury, especially one during the previous four to six hours, should be taken to surgery. For remote injuries in which suppuration has already taken place, heat, rest, and elevation are indicated, with possible drainage of any collections of pus which may have formed.

SURGERY

Treatment within the operating room (figure 1–3 and figure 1–4) should proceed in this order:
1. Pneumatic cuff tourniquet
2. Anesthesia (block or general)
3. Preparation of injured part, in this order:
   Detergent scrub of surrounding skin
   Gentle detergent cleansing of wound
   Normal saline irrigation of wound, large amount
   Repetition of same procedure (scrubbing, cleansing, irrigation) with new setup
4. Limited debridement with head loupe magnification (figure 1–5)
5. Identification of injured structures
6. Procedure DEPENDENT UPON TYPE OF CASE:

Recent injury seen early Clean wound Little trauma Operator skilled, interested, and rested	DEFINITIVE SURGERY to be done at time of original debridement, including tendon repair, nerve repair, and skin grafting.
Injury seen late Operator unfamiliar Severe trauma Much contamination	SKIN CLOSURE ONLY, FOR PRIMARY HEALING—OR CLEANSED WOUND COVERED with sterile gauze moistened with antibiotic solution (delayed emergency). DEFINITIVE SURGERY DELAYED 3 to 6 weeks for deep structures.
Bite wounds whenever seen Blast wounds whenever seen Gunshot wounds whenever seen	DEBRIDEMENT ONLY. LEAVE OPEN.

The use of a pneumatic cuff tourniquet is important to properly identify and avoid further injury to the small structures involved.

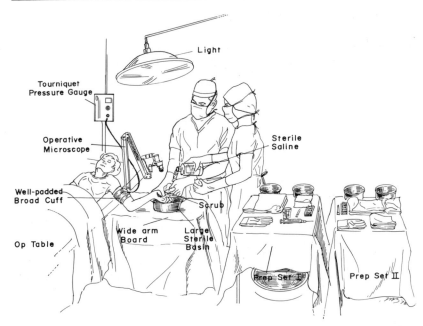

Figure 1–3. The operating room equipped for the treatment of hand injuries. Shaving and extensive cleansing of the skin of the forearm and hand with soap and detergent combined with copious irrigation of the wound, both carried out in two stages, is the first responsibility in order to avoid infection and to promote early primary healing. A large sterile basin under the hand is a simple way to catch the irrigation fluid. Although primary repair of tendons and nerves can be attended to in ideal cases at this time, it can usually be done later, through new incisions, with less chance of infection.

Anesthesia may be either local or general. In the preparation of the injured part, the surrounding skin should be thoroughly cleansed and the wound itself irrigated with a gentle detergent and normal saline solution. Fingernails of the injured hand should be cut short to remove dirt. It has been customary in my clinical experience to have the setup made in two stages so that after the cleansing has proceeded to a certain point and the wound irrigated, the identical procedure is then repeated with a second sterile setup, following which sterile drapes are applied. Next, using head loupe magnification and a pneumatic cuff tourniquet, limited debridement to preserve important structures is carried out (figure 1–5). *Debridement* means wound excision and removal of foreign bodies. (As originally used by the French it meant enlargement of the wound for removal of foreign bodies and drainage.[2] The English meaning of debridement as it is used today came about during the First World War, 1914–1918.)

However, the hand, with so many closely packed, important structures, does not allow wide wound excision; instead, devitalized tissues only are removed, preserving as many important structures as possible.

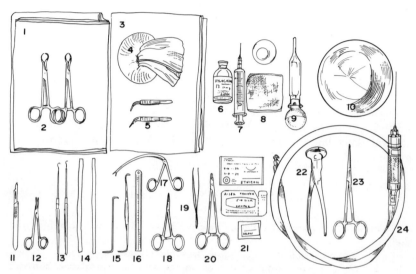

Figure 1–4. Instruments used in the treatment of hand injuries. 1 and 3, drapes 2, towel clips 4, stockinette 5, vascular clamps 6 and 7, local anesthetic 8, gauze 9, irrigating syringe 10, basin 11, scalpel 12, small sharp scissors (several sizes and shapes) 13, skin hooks 14, rubber drains 15, retractors 16, metal scale 17, tendon threading forceps 18, fine hemostats 19, fine pick-up forceps 20, needle holder 21, sutures (tendon and otherwise) 22, Kirschner wire cutter 23, heavy clamp for bone 24, motor drill and Kirschner wire. Fine instruments for work under the microscope should be made available for nerve repair.

After limited debridement, the decision must be made whether or not definitive surgery is to be done at this time. As indicated (in the block within the surgery outline), the case seen early after injury which has been traumatized with a sharp instrument should be taken care of definitively, if the operator is skilled and interested in this type of work. If the case is seen late—more than a few hours after injury—or if the operator is unfamiliar with the techniques of tendon and nerve surgery, it is perfectly permissible and undoubtedly better only to carry out adequate skin closure of the soft tissues after the debridement rather than to attempt to proceed with repairs with which the operator is not too familiar. It should be emphasized that definitive surgery both for tendon repair and nerve repair can well be performed three to six weeks later, after the wound has healed. A new aseptic incision then can be made with less chance of infection. This can be scheduled as elective surgery with an operator who is interested and experienced in this type of work. Fractures, however, should be reduced and immobilized at the earliest possible time. Like debridement, this should be taken care of on the day of injury if at all possible.

Delayed primary wound closure (see chapter 4 also) with definitive repair of tendons and nerves through the original wound one to several days after injury has been advocated by Iselin[6] and Madsen.[7] This method of treatment is also called delayed emergency. The wound should be cleansed and debrided at the earliest possible time after injury and covered with sterile gauze moistened with antibiotic solution, such as 0.5% neomycin, 0.1% chloramphenicol, or bacitracin 250–1000 units per ml. Although Madsen has repaired tendons several days later, I have delayed tendon repair only twenty-four hours.

SPECIAL FEATURES OF THE HAND

Features of the hand which must be considered when treating injuries to it are:

1. The presence of small structures closely arranged
2. The delicate nature of nerves, joints, and tendon gliding surfaces (all readily injured by trauma)
3. The low resistance to infection
4. The importance of normal sensation to hand function
5. The importance of mobility of the parts normally. Interferences to normal movement are:
     open wounds
     edema
     cicatrix

The physician does not have control over the severity of the original injury but should assume the responsibility of not adding to it.

The great mobility of the many small joints of the fingers and thumb as well as the exquisite sensitivity of the digits must be emphasized as of the greatest importance to preserve and to restore, since the normal dexterity of the hand depends upon both. All joints of the body stiffen when immobilized. This is especially true of the fifteen small joints of the digits. Hence, every effort should be made to keep these joints moving to prevent stiffening (see chapter 4).

TOURNIQUET

Bleeding from incision through living tissues has two adverse effects locally, from the surgeon's standpoint. First, it obscures the

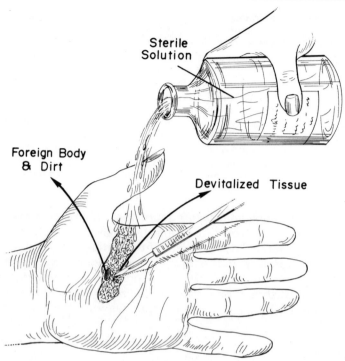

Figure 1−5. Debridement: the surgeon's effort to convert a contaminated wound into a clean wound. The cleansing and irrigation are done in two stages prior to draping and removal of devitalized tissues is done after sterile draping. Foreign bodies are always looked for in the wound.

operative field. Second, it stains the tissues red. Both of these factors interfere with visualization and identification of small anatomical structures in the wound. The careful operator clamps vessels before dividing them for this reason as well as to diminish blood loss.

In the extremities, the blood flow can be stopped by physical proximal constriction. For surgical purposes, if the vessels are emptied prior to application of the constricting mechanism, the operator has the advantage of dividing and cutting tissues in a bloodless field which allows much more accurate identification and manipulation than is possible when the blood is flowing. In working with the hand this is very desirable.

The adverse effects of stopping the blood flow are:

   1. Pressure phenomena in the area of constriction if this is too severe

   2. Metabolic alteration in the tissues distal to the constriction

These factors are controlled by guarding the amount and evenness of the force applied and by limiting the length of time of its application.

Historically, tourniquets have been used to stop the blood flow in extremities since the second century A.D. They were of two types—temporary and permanent—amputation was carried out just distal to the latter. Esmarch,[4] in 1872, advocated wrapping the arm with a broad rubber bandage to empty the blood vessels prior to applying the temporary constricting rubber band proximal. This technique with a proximal pneumatic cuff is still utilized today in most clinics for hand surgery. Harvey Cushing[3] was the first to advocate the use of the pneumatic tourniquet for operations on the arm. Having been asked to care for patients with tourniquet paralysis, he was seeking a device with evenly controlled pressure that could be applied, removed, and reapplied at will during the course of an operation, thus greatly increasing the safety of the technique. He cautioned against high pressure on the nerves at the site of constriction as well as prolonged interruption of blood flow.

The use of a pneumatic cuff tourniquet during primary wound treatment today is advocated so that fine delicate structures can be more readily identified and protected from further injury. A broad cuff should be chosen and the upper arm wrapped with protective padding, so that the force of the cuff pressure is evenly distributed (figure 1–6). It should be inflated to between 250 and 300 mm Hg and can be left in place for ninety minutes with a great margin of

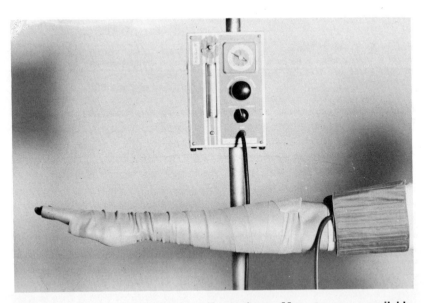

Figure 1–6. The broad pneumatic cuff tourniquet. Many types are available. The distal portion of the extremity is wrapped snugly with a broad elastic bandage to empty the blood vessels before the cuff is inflated. The elastic bandage is then completely removed. This procedure is usually carried out after the arm is prepped and sterile drapes applied.

safety. Many operators leave it in place longer, but I advocate a ninety-minute limit because of my own clinical experience and the experimental work cited in the following paragraph.

If a longer period of time is required, the cuff can be temporarily deflated and reapplied after ten to fifteen minutes of blood flow. Solonen et al.[12] and, more recently, Wilgis[13] have monitored pH, Po_2, and Pco_2 during tourniquet ischemia. The pH dropped to markedly acidotic levels at two hours; concomitantly the Po_2 reduced precipitously after one-half hour and then slowed to almost immeasurable levels after two hours. The Pco_2 increased at a progressive rate. These studies substantiate the wisdom of limiting blood flow-interruption to the shortest possible time. Paletta et al.[11] have shown that hypothermia and intravenous heparin diminish the adverse effects of tourniquet ischemia in the dog, but this is difficult to utilize in man.

To judge from these observations, clinical experience, and the work of Bruner[1] and others, it is best to keep tourniquet ischemia time to about ninety minutes. If this is done and the cuff is broad

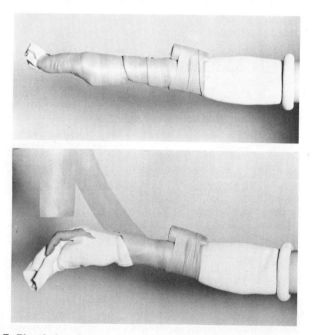

Figure 1–7. Elastic bandage wrapped with slight overlaps, the distal portion only being unraveled. This gives a bloodless field distally for short procedures (a method originally used by Esmarch).[4] It does not have the same safety as the pneumatic cuff.

and well padded, it is a boon to hand surgery and should be used during the primary treatment of hand wounds as well as in elective surgery. The gauge should be checked periodically to detect any inaccuracies, since the safety of the device depends upon the cuff pressure not exceeding 250 to 300 mm Hg.

For short procedures the elastic bandage[4] may be wrapped centripetally and the peripheral portion removed while the proximal portion still shuts off the blood supply from the area being operated (figure 1–7). This is not advocated for long procedures and is not considered to have the same safety factors as the pneumatic tourniquet.

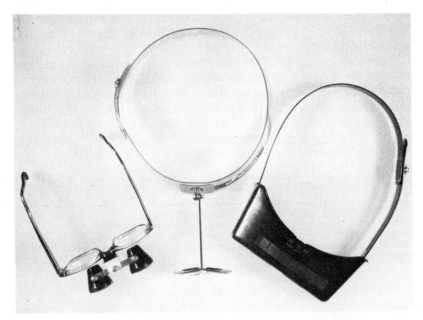

Figure 1–8. Head loupes. These ocular loupes with a magnification of about two diameters are a great aid during debridement of wounds of the hand.

MAGNIFICATION

Magnification is also useful to prevent further injury. The operative microscope with its higher magnification is rather cumbersome when working with large wounds because of its size and the small area of its field. Newer models are being developed which are more adaptable for upper extremity work. I prefer a head loupe (figure 1 –8) with a magnification of two diameters when dealing with a large area. This is useful for manipulation, identification, and repair of structures, as well as for wound debridement. It can readily be used but is easily moved out of the line of vision when not needed. A microscope can be brought into a small area of the large field for a specific purpose (see chapter 9). This method of utilization prevents "tubular vision."

WOUNDS REQUIRING SPECIAL ATTENTION

Gunshot (Bullet) Wounds

Bullets tear through tissues at all levels, producing destruction in their path. The amount of damage produced depends on many variables, including the weight, design, flight pattern, and especially the velocity of the bullet. This velocity to a large extent determines the size of the area of destruction about the bullet track.

Most bullet wounds encountered in civilian practice are termed low-velocity (less than 1,800 feet per second).[17] Even these do extensive damage in the track of the bullet, although the cross-section size of the damage area is not as great as in the case of the high-velocity missile.

As the bullet strikes the skin, it carries organisms from the surface and bits of any clothing in with it, both of which may become deeply embedded. These, along with the devitalized tissues produced in the bullet track, make conditions ideal for infection. For this reason, it is my opinion that bullet wounds should be treated surgically, especially if an important structure such as an artery, joint, or tendon sheath has been injured. If no important deep structure has been injured, expectant treatment with systemic antibiotics may be employed. The arguments pro and con are given by several authors.[18, 19, 20, 21]

When important deep structures are injured, the wound should be excised at either end and explored as completely as possible for foreign bodies. Devitalized tissues should be removed, and thorough irrigation with normal saline should be carried out. The wound should then be left open and systemic antibiotics as well as local antibiotics, such as 0.5% neomycin, placed in the wound to inhibit bacterial growth.

If a joint is penetrated, the track should be left open down to the joint until the danger of infection is past, usually in three to five days. Secondary closure can then be carried out.

In the case of important blood vessel injury, the vessel should be repaired and placed away from the bullet track if possible, leaving the wound open to be treated with antibiotics. The bullet, which is a foreign body, should be removed during the debridement if at all feasible.

Shotgun Wounds

In shotgun wounds at close range there is considerable blast effect which damages the tissues deeply. Since the limit of this damage is hard to recognize, repeated excision of devitalized tissue at intervals of several days may be necessary to get a clean wound bed which will heal without infection if skin is grafted or the wound closed secondarily.

Shell Fragment Wounds

Metal fragments act as foreign bodies if left in the tissues. There is much fibrotic reaction about them with time. This may cause continued discomfort to the patient. Recurrent infection about retained metal fragments is also common. For this reason, like bullets or other foreign bodies, it is best to remove them at the original debridement if at all possible. The wounds should be left open at primary treatment and closed secondarily after the danger of infection has passed.

Injection Injury (Grease, Paint, etc.)

High-pressure grease guns and paint sprayers can inject their contents through the skin and inflate the entire subcutaneous tissues of a finger or the palm. This diffuses irritant foreign material containing microorganisms throughout the tissues. The injected material is insinuated between all parts of the injected tissue and is very difficult to remove.

Treatment should be early wide incision, excision, and cleansing. The task is tremendously difficult but should be tackled as soon as possible. The situation only worsens with time. Severe cases may require amputation of the part. Early evacuation may avoid this. Figure 1–9 shows the right index finger of a twenty-year-old man who was first seen forty-eight hours after injury. Partial amputation was necessary. No immediate evacuation of the material had been performed.

Human Bite

Because of the many microorganisms present in the mouth, including spirochetes, fusiform bacilli, and streptococci, human bite

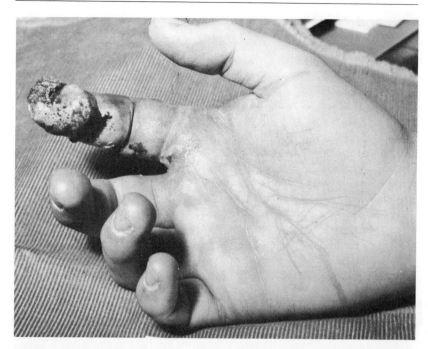

Figure 1–9. The right hand of a workman who accidentally discharged a paint sprayer against the tip of his index finger two days earlier. The entire finger had been "inflated" with paint. Gangrene of the end of the finger has occurred requiring amputation through the proximal phalanx. Immediate wide excision of the foreign material might have saved more of the finger.

wounds are serious and carry a very high rate of infection. Often the history will not be given accurately. All puncture wounds about the knuckles should be held in suspicion as impalement wounds on teeth while fighting. These have grave potential for infection. A tooth is readily driven through the skin, extensor hood, and into the metacarpophalangeal (M-P) joint space. When the finger is straightened, the tissues shift and the joint is sealed off.

Treatment should consist of extensive cleansing of the surrounding area, debridement, removal of foreign bodies, and copious irrigation of the wound with normal saline. The wound should be left open, no deep repair attempted, and if joint or tendon sheath has been entered, antibiotics (such as erythromycin, sodium oxacillin, or penicillin) should be given until the danger of infection has passed. Tetanus immunization should be included. Secondary closure should be done when necessary. The patient should be followed closely for several days because serious infection can develop rapidly.

Dog and Wild Animal Bite

The potential for infection from animal bite wounds is similar to human bite wounds, and the same wound treatment and precautions are indicated, including tetanus immunization. In addition to this, the danger of rabies demands that the animal be under quarantine-observation for ten days to determine whether it has transmissible disease. The local wound should be extensively cleaned and debrided and left open. In the case of a bite by a known rabid animal, the use of fuming nitric acid in the wound to destroy virus, although controversial, is probably still wise—but only under these circumstances. Also, if the animal is known to be rabid or dies during the ten-day observation period, immunization must be started at once. This should consist of rabies hyperimmune serum (passive immunization) followed by a course of rabies killed virus duck embryo vaccine given daily for at least fourteen doses.

The risk of a bite from an unknown stray or wild animal poses a serious problem. The risk of rabies in the community must be considered. Usually the best solution is to give prophylactic treatment.

Cat Bite

The danger of bacterial infection from cat bite is significant. Many different organisms may be present. *Pasteurella multocida,* a frequent inhabitant of the oral cavity of the cat, can produce serious cellulitis and osteomyelitis, but is fortunately sensitive to penicillin.

These wounds should be carefully cleansed and debrided, as described earlier, and tetanus toxoid and prophylactic antibiotics given.

Cat-Scratch Fever

Cat-scratch fever, thought to have a viral etiology, must be differentiated from bacterial cellulitis. Lymphadenopathy may be marked. Culture the wound exudate, if present. Antibiotics should be given to overcome coexisting microorganisms.

Snake Bite

Most snake bites occur on the extremities; about one-third of these occur on the upper extremity, the hand being a frequent site, especially in children.

The venom of poisonous snakes can produce death or severe local destruction of tissue because of the neurotoxins and hemolysins which it contains. Snyder, Straight, and Glenn[16] have outlined treatment on the basis of ninety-six poisonous bites they have attended. Methods of prevention are outlined, and in dangerous parts of the country they recommend carrying a "snake bite kit" which includes a tourniquet, scalpel, polyvalent antivenin (Wyeth), and 100 mgm hydrocortisone sodium succinate. Emergency treatment of poisonous snake bite in the field should include:

1. Avoidance of exertion and excitement
2. Identification of the snake
3. Application of a tourniquet proximal to the bite to obstruct venous return
4. Incision of the fang marks
5. Immobilization of the part
6. Venom neutralization locally and systemically at earliest possible time with polyvalent antivenin (Wyeth), after testing for horse serum sensitivity

The patient should be admitted to the hospital for careful observation and complete study. Blood counts, bleeding and clotting times, prothrombin time, sedimentation rate, electrolyte concentrations, and electrocardiograph should be obtained. Antivenin should be instituted or continued. Respiratory and circulatory complications must be treated actively. Local excision of the tissue about the fang marks may remove some venom if done early. Tetanus toxoid and antibiotics should be given prophylactically.

Spider Bite

Nearly all spiders are venomous.[14, 15] The ability to inject and the amount of venom injected, although usually less than that of venomous snakes, can be dangerous—especially that of the black widow spider (*Latrodectus mactans*). Antivenin exists and may be available. Children and victims with nausea, cramps, muscle pains, or headache should be hospitalized. Elevation of blood pressure may occur.

The bite of the brown recluse spider (*Loxosceles reclusa*) may produce fever, nausea, malaise, and significant necrosis at the site of envenomation. This arthropod, so-named because of its tendency to stay hidden, is recognized by a violin-shaped marking on its dorsal cephalothorax. Local and systemic corticosteroids are recommended as well as local excision of the bite area.

Washing Machine and Industrial Roller Injury

The turning rolls of a clothes wringer constitute a hazard to the operator. Any slight distraction may cause the hand to be caught and drawn in along with the clothes. When this happens, the width between the rolls and the suddenness with which the safety release is activated determines the severity of the injury. Unfortunately, many victims are children who are not able to release themselves. Figure 1–10 shows the right hand of a two-and-one-half-year-old child who was caught between the turning rolls of his deaf mother's washing machine for an unknown time-interval, probably twenty or thirty minutes. She was outside hanging up clothes and could not hear his screams.

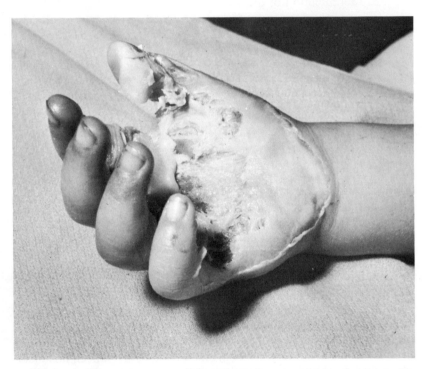

Figure 1–10. Right hand of a two-and-a-half-year-old boy caught in his mother's clothes wringer for twenty or thirty minutes. There was severe friction burn of the palm in addition to avulsion of the skin. The blood vessels in the palm were coagulated and all digits except the base of the thumb were lost in spite of all treatment.

The case was extreme. There was charring of the tissues of the palm with impairment of circulation of the fingers and thumb at the time he was first seen. In spite of all treatment, including stellate blocks and dextran, it was not possible to restore circulation to the digits; they were lost, with the exception of a portion of the base of the thumb.

The diagnosis of wringer injury is usually made by history. Determination of the extent of the injury is much more difficult when first seen.

The following factors are helpful in deciding how severe the injury is:

1. Length of time in the mechanism
2. Amount of edema or hematoma
3. Presence of abrasions, lacerations, or avulsions
4. Presence of charring of the skin
5. Circulation (color, presence of pulses)
6. Presence of fractures (not frequent)

It is safest to admit all but the mildest cases to the hospital since deep injury may be much more severe than appears on the surface. Treatment for washing machine or roller injury should follow this order:

1. X-ray, although fractures are not common.
2. Gently cleanse the skin with detergent.
3. Irrigate with saline and debride open wounds.
4. Close wound loosely. Beware of the circulation in reverse flaps; cover with free skin graft or pedicle flap if necessary, except in the face of severe contamination.
5. With severe contamination, leave the wound open after after cleansing and debridement. Use local and systemic antibiotics.
6. Reduce any existing fractures. Splint in position of function.
7. Apply gentle pressure dressing with fingertips visible for observation of circulation.
8. Give dextran intravenously and stellate blocks to improve circulation.
9. Drain large hematomas.
10. Continue observation.
11. Follow up with skin grafting (free graft or pedicle flap), as required.
12. Keep joints supple.

Fractures are uncommon since the compression force is applied equally on both sides. Angulation during efforts at extraction may cause fractures. Tetanus toxoid and antibiotics should be used when contaminated open wounds are present.

Industrial rollers of many types are in use which offer similar or even greater hazard to the workman's hands and arms. Many of these have steel rolls which exert tremendous forces, and some are hot, combining burn with severe crush injury. Treatment must be individualized, but in general it is similar to the washing machine wringer injury treatment described here.

Finger-Ring Injury

Finger rings create a hazard by catching on nails and other projections. The entire weight or momentum of the body may be transferred to the small metal band about the base of the finger with dire results. The injuries are serious. The looser the ring, the greater the hazard; the sharper its edges, the more likely it is to cut. The entire skin may be avulsed from the finger. The skin and tendons may be divided or the entire finger may be torn away, as happened to a young executive who jumped from a platform while examining the warehouse of his company. A ring he was wearing on his small finger caught on a hook in the wall and transferred his entire body

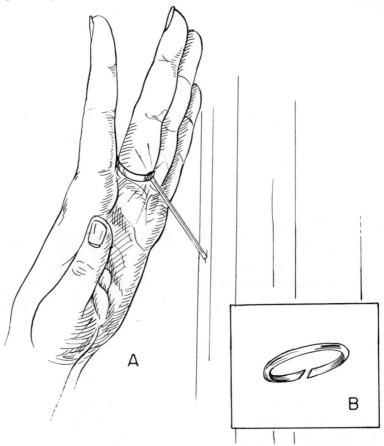

Figure 1–11. Finger-ring injury. *A*, the ring catches on a nail or hook as the patient jumps from a platform or other object transferring the full force of the body to the finger ring. The ring may tear off the skin of the finger, cut the tendons, fracture the bones, or tear off the finger completely. *B*, a safety modification (split ring) which was recommended by Frackelton and works if the ring is not strong.

weight to his small finger, which was torn off. Figure 1−11 shows the hazard diagrammatically.

Workmen are best advised not to wear finger rings. Frackelton has advised a split ring which will bend (see figure 1−11*B*).

Since the injuries vary greatly, treatment must be individualized. Complete avulsion of the skin must be covered by free grafting and/or a pedicle flap. Tendons and nerves should be repaired and fractures stabilized. Lacerations of soft tissues should be sutured back into place if flaps are viable.

Bibliography

PROCEDURE
1. Bruner, Julian M.: Safety factors in the use of the pneumatic tourniquet for hemostasis in surgery of the hand, J. Bone Joint Surg. 33-A: 221−24, 1951.
2. Colwill, John C.: Introduction, in Iselin, Mark: *Atlas of Hand Surgery*, p. vii (New York: McGraw-Hill Book Co., 1964).
3. Cushing, Harvey: Pneumatic tourniquets: With especial reference to their use in craniotomies, Medical News 84: 577−80, 1904.
4. Esmarch, Friedrich von, and Kowalzig, E.: *Surgical Technic*, trans. Grau, Ludwig H., and Sullivan, William N.; ed. Senn, Nicholas, p. 225 (New York: Macmillan Co., 1901).
5. Hinman, Frank, Jr.: The rational use of tourniquets, Int. Abstr. Surg. 81: 357−66, 1945.
6. Iselin, M.: "Delayed emergency" in fresh wounds of the hand, Proc. R. Soc. Med. 51: 713−14, 1958.
7. Madsen, Erin: Delayed primary suture of flexor tendons cut in the digital sheath, J. Bone Joint Surg. 52-B: 264−67, 1970.
8. Moberg, Erik: Objective methods of determining the functional value of sensibility in the hand, J. Bone Joint Surg. 40-B: 454−76, 1958.
9. Önne, Lars: Recovery of sensibility and sudomotor activity in the hand after nerve suture, Acta Chir. Scand. Suppl. 300: 1−69, 1962.
10. Paletta, Francis X.; Willman, Vallee; and Ship, Arthur G.: Prolonged tourniquet ischemia of extremities, J. Bone Joint Surg. 42-A: 945−50, 1960.
11. Paletta, F. X.; Shehadi, Sameer I.; Mudd, J. G.; and Cooper, T.: Hypothermia and tourniquet ischemia, Plast. Reconstr. Surg. 29: 531−38, 1962.
12. Solonen, Kauko A.; Tarkkanen, Leena; Närvänen, Sakari; and Gordin, Ruben: Metabolic changes in the upper limb during

tourniquet ischaemia: A clinical study, Acta Orthop. Scand. 39:20–32, 1968.

13. Wilgis, E. F. Shaw: Observations on the effects of tourniquet ischemia, J. Bone Joint Surg. 53-A:1343–46, 1971.

BITE WOUNDS
14. Asel, Norman D.: Spider bites (*Loxosceles reclusa*), in Conn, Howard F. (ed.): *Current Therapy*, p. 880 (Philadelphia: W. B. Saunders Co., 1969).
15. Russell, Findlay E.: Bites of spiders and other arthropods, in Conn, Howard F. (ed.): *Current Therapy*, pp. 878–79 (Philadelphia: W. B. Saunders Co., 1969).
16. Snyder, Clifford C.; Straight, Richard; and Glenn, James: The snakebitten hand, Plast. Reconstr. Surg. 49:275–82, 1972.

GUNSHOT WOUNDS
17. DeMuth, W. E., Jr., and Smith, J. M.: High-velocity bullet wounds of muscle and bone: The basis of rational early treatment, J. Trauma 6:744–55, 1966.
18. Dziemian, Arthur J.; Mendelson, Janice A.; and Lindsey, Douglas: Comparison of the wounding characteristics of some commonly encountered bullets, J. Trauma 1:341–53, 1961.
19. Hampton, Oscar P., Jr.: The indications for debridement of gunshot (bullet) wounds of the extremities in civilian practice, J. Trauma 1:368–72, 1961.
20. Morgan, Milton M.; Spencer, Andrew D.; and Hershey, Falls B.: Debridement of civilian gunshot wounds of soft tissue, J. Trauma 1:354–60, 1961.
21. Ziperman, H. Haskell: The management of soft tissue missile wounds in war and peace, J. Trauma 1:361–67, 1961.

ROLLER INJURY
22. Iritani, Roy I., and Siler, Vinton E.: Wringer injuries of the upper extremity, Surg. Gynecol. Obstet. 113:677–80, 1961.

CHAPTER 2

Anesthesia

ABSTRACT

General anesthesia is justifiable for extensive operations on the hand, especially if grafts must be taken from another part of the body. Anesthesia of the upper extremity may be provided by blocking the major nerves at various levels as outlined on the following pages. Nerve blocks have the advantage of safety, especially when the patient has recently eaten. The surgeon can administer the more peripheral blocks if he wishes after the field has been prepared for surgery. Regional intravenous block is also described.

Pitfalls

1. *Aspiration of stomach contents into the lungs if general anesthesia is given with food in the stomach*
2. *Hypersensitivity to the local anesthetic agent utilized*
3. *Intravascular injection of a local anesthetic*
4. *Unsuccessful nerve block*
5. *Pneumothorax following supraclavicular brachial block*
6. *Vascular spasm of digital vessels if vasoconstrictors are utilized in anesthetic agents injected beyond the wrist level*
7. *Possible nerve injury if more than two milliliters of anesthetic are injected within a nerve sheath*

The use of general anesthesia for operations upon the upper extremity is quite justifiable under most circumstances, especially when the length of the procedure is uncertain or expected to be great. Also it is the method of choice when additional areas of the body other than one extremity must be anesthetized. Its use, however, requires the presence of an anesthesiologist, who may not always be available. Since injuries may occur at any time and human beings eat frequently, it is not uncommon to encounter an injured patient with a full stomach. This greatly increases the risk of general anesthesia.

The anatomy of the upper extremity allows the blockade of the main nerve trunks with local anesthetics at many locations along their routes, as shown in figure 2-1. These blocks may also be desirable for certain patients with systemic diseases, especially cardiorespiratory conditions which increase the risk of general

41

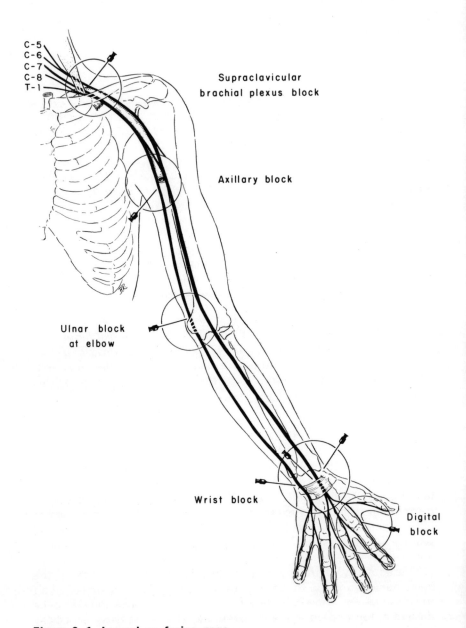

C-5
C-6
C-7
C-8
T-1

Supraclavicular
brachial plexus block

Axillary block

Ulnar block
at elbow

Wrist block

Digital
block

Figure 2–1. Legend on facing page.

anesthesia. The intravenous instillation of lidocaine distal to an inflated tourniquet after emptying all vessels of their blood by wrapping the extremity tightly with an elastic bandage has also proven to be a sure method of anesthesia in the extremity. These techniques are given on the following pages.

SUPRACLAVICULAR BRACHIAL PLEXUS BLOCK

With the supraclavicular approach, the anesthetic needle is inserted through the posterior triangle of the neck, about two centimeters above the midportion of the clavicle, just posterior to the posterior border of the anterior scalene muscle, which is palpated when the patient raises his head. The subclavian artery is palpated as it passes under the clavicle and over the first rib just posterior to the scalenus anticus muscle (figure 2–1). The anesthetic solution of choice (30 ml of 1% lidocaine works well) is injected through a $1\frac{1}{2}$-inch 22-gauge needle just posterior to the artery, about the trunks and divisions of the brachial plexus as they pass over the same structure. Paresthesias in the hand are a good guide to the proper position of the needle prior to injection.

Pneumothorax is a possible complication. Care should be taken to direct the needle against the first rib just posterior to the subclavian artery to avoid this. In case of shortness of breath after the block, this complication should be suspected.

AXILLARY BLOCK

The patient should be lying down with the arm abducted to 90°, the elbow flexed, and the forearm rotated dorsally onto a pillow. A rubber tourniquet is placed snugly about the arm just beyond the axillary fold to direct the anesthetic solution centrally toward the brachial plexus.

The skin central to the tourniquet is cleansed with antiseptic

Figure 2–1. Nerve blocks of the upper extremity. The upper part of the diagram shows supraclavicular brachial plexus block. For supraclavicular brachial plexus block, the anesthetic solution is injected into and about the trunks and divisions of the brachial plexus, as shown by the top needle. A point just posterior to the scalenus anticus muscle and the subclavian artery, about 2 cm above the midportion of the clavicle, is chosen for the injection. Aspirate frequently to avoid intravascular injection. The other needles indicate additional levels at which conduction of the nerves of the upper extremity may be interrupted by the injection of anesthetic solutions.

solution and, using sterile technique, a 1-inch 24-gauge needle is inserted vertically toward the humerus into the fascial compartment containing the brachial artery and the median, ulnar, and radial nerves as they emerge from the brachial plexus (figure 2–2). The pulsations of the brachial artery are a guide during insertion of the needle and during injection of the anesthetic solution about it. The needle should pulsate with the artery prior to injection to be sure it is within the proper fascial space. Twenty-five milliliters of anesthetic solution, such as 1% lidocaine, are injected about the brachial artery and the nerves. Intermittent aspiration will prevent intravascular injection.

This more peripheral site of block avoids the risk of pneumothorax.

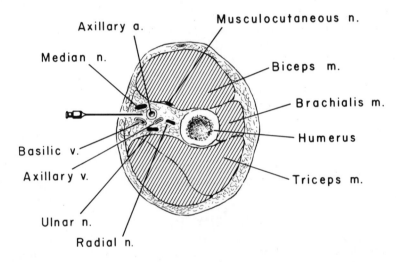

Figure 2–2. Axillary block. With the patient lying down and with the arm abducted to 90°, the elbow flexed, and the forearm rotated dorsally on a pillow, the anesthetic solution is injected into the fascial compartment containing the brachial artery and nerves. Aspirate frequently to avoid intravascular injection.

The humerus is used as a backstop instead of the first rib.[8] Its success rate has been 90 percent in the hands of Kasdan et al.[7]

ULNAR NERVE BLOCK AT ELBOW

The very superficial position of the ulnar nerve as it passes below the medial epicondyle of the humerus at the elbow offers an excellent site for the injection of local anesthetic agents (figure 2–3).

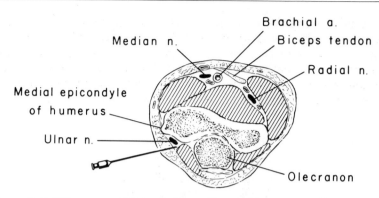

Figure 2–3. Ulnar nerve block at elbow. The ulnar nerve is palpated behind the medial epicondyle of the humerus, and 8–10 ml of anesthetic solution such as 1% lidocaine injected about it with a 24-gauge needle.

The nerve can be palpated and held with the finger as 8 to 10 ml of 1% lidocaine or other agent is injected through a 1½-inch 24-gauge needle into and about it. A paresthesia is desirable, indicating that the needle point is present in the nerve proper. One or two milliliters are injected here, and the balance then injected about the nerve by altering the position of the needle slightly. This gives an excellent block of the ulnar border of the hand. When combined with median and radial nerve blockade at the wrist, complete anesthesia of the hand is obtained.

WRIST BLOCK

The wrist block (figure 2–4) is excellent when the surgeon is working alone on short procedures. It is quite practical because the injections are given in the field already prepared for surgery. The tourniquet on the upper arm should be inflated after the anesthetic is given. Usually the patient is comfortable for twenty to forty minutes, and during this time much important dissection can be carried out. The operation is then completed with the blood flowing.

Median Nerve Block at Wrist

The median nerve lies superficial to the sublimis flexors of the long and ring fingers on the volar surface of the wrist. The palmaris longus tendon, when present, lies superficial to the median nerve and slightly to its ulnar side. This location is essentially the middle of the wrist when viewed from the volar aspect. A 1-inch 22- or 24-gauge needle is inserted through a skin wheal in a vertical

direction. An attempt is made to obtain a paresthesia radiating to
the thumb, index, or long finger. If so, a few milliliters of 1% lidocaine are injected here. The needle is then slightly withdrawn and
directed toward the palm and advanced several centimeters, where
the balance of 10 ml of the anesthetic solution is injected into the
flexor compartment beneath the transverse carpal ligament. If a

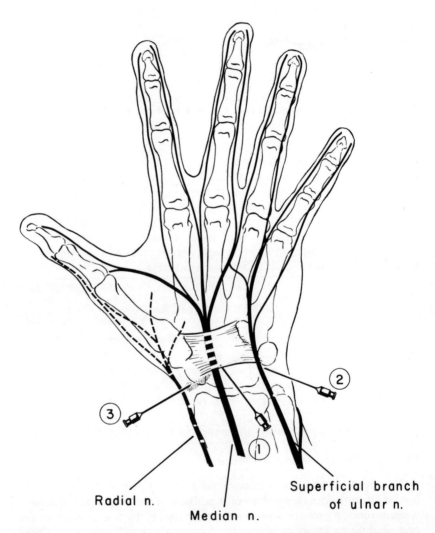

Radial n.

Median n.

Superficial branch
of ulnar n.

**Figure 2–4. Wrist block. Anesthetic solution is placed directly about the
median and ulnar nerves and injected subcutaneously to encircle the wrist
(see text).**

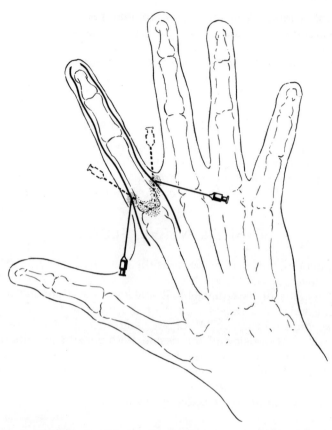

Figure 2–5. Digital nerve block. The anesthetic solution is injected with a 24- or 26-gauge needle about the volar and dorsal aspects of the hand, in a V-shaped manner, at the base of the digit to be anesthetized. The subcutaneous tissues are infiltrated and the digital nerves are surrounded with anesthetic solution without compressing the blood vessels. Vasoconstrictors should not be used here. For surgery on the finger after the anesthetic is administered, a Penrose drain can be used to provide a bloodless field, as shown in the digital Allen test (figure 4–9, page 82).

22-gauge needle is utilized, the tissues of the palm can be seen to distend slightly as the injection is made.

Ulnar Nerve Block at Wrist

As well as at the elbow (page 45), the ulnar nerve can also be injected in its fascial compartment just radial to the pisiform bone. Several milliliters of anesthetic solution is placed in the nerve after paresthesia, the same as for the ulnar nerve block at the elbow, and

4 to 6 ml is injected in the fascial compartment about it.

The elbow block of the ulnar nerve has the advantage of complete blockade of all elements to the hand. The wrist block at the pisiform leaves the rather large dorsal sensory branch to the back of the hand unanesthetized. This must be blocked by the subcutaneous infiltration described next.

Radial Nerve and Dorsal Branch of Ulnar Nerve Wrist Block

The wrist block is completed by circumferential subcutaneous injection of 10 ml of 1% lidocaine, which blocks the dorsal branch of the ulnar nerve, the terminal branches of the radial styloid, as well as the terminal filaments from the dorsal nerves of the forearm.

DIGITAL NERVE BLOCK

The digital nerve block is perhaps the most frequently used nerve block. It gives excellent anesthesia of the entire digit. About 10 ml of 1% lidocaine or its equivalent is injected in a V-shaped manner about the volar and dorsal aspect of the hand at the base of the particular digit through a 24- or 26-gauge needle. This site of injection allows distension of the tissues with anesthetic solution but without constriction (figure 2—5).

Particular attention is given to the volar digital nerves which enter the digit anterolaterally on its volar surface. No vasoconstrictor should be utilized in the solution at this level.

STELLATE GANGLION BLOCK

Anesthetic blockade of the sympathetic nerve supply of the upper extremity, usually for the relief of vascular spasm or pain, can be accomplished specifically by anesthetizing the sympathetic chain in the region of the stellate ganglion at the base of the neck. The block is best carried out in the operative suite. One of the simplest approaches is by the anterior or paratracheal route. With the patient lying down, head extended, and the head of the table elevated, the sulcus between the trachea and the carotid sheath is palpated with the finger, one inch above the sternoclavicular junction (figure 2—6). A 1½-inch 24-gauge needle is advanced vertically through the sulcus adjacent to the palpating finger to the anterior surface of the seventh cervical vertebra and then withdrawn one-quarter of an inch. Ten milliliters of 1% lidocaine or other suitable anesthetic is injected here. Hoarseness from recurrent laryngeal blockade is common. Only

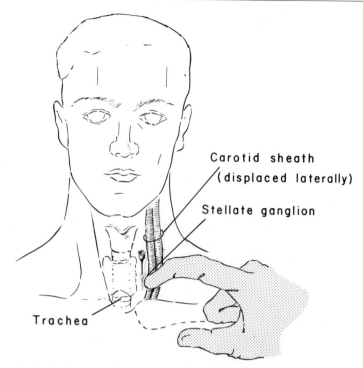

Carotid sheath
(displaced laterally)

Stellate ganglion

Trachea

Figure 2–6. Stellate ganglion block. The patient should be lying down with chin up, and the head of the table should be elevated moderately. The carotid sheath is displaced laterally with the index finger. The needle is introduced vertically through the skin and deeper tissues to the transverse process of the seventh cervical vertebra and withdrawn one-fourth inch. Ten milliliters of 1% lidocaine or similar anesthetic are injected slowly. Aspirate intermittently to avoid intravascular injection.

one side should be injected at any time. Enophthalmos, miosis, and injection of the scleral vessels indicate a successful block with its desired vascular dilatations. The temperature of the patient's hand should rise on the side of the block because of increased blood flow, and the skin should become dry because of interruption of the nerve supply to the sweat glands.

Any peripheral nerve block gives a similar effect because the sympathetic nerve fibers travel within the peripheral nerves.

INTRAVENOUS REGIONAL ANESTHESIA

Bier[3] in 1908 produced regional anesthesia by injecting a local anesthetic agent intravenously into a bloodless extremity distal to a

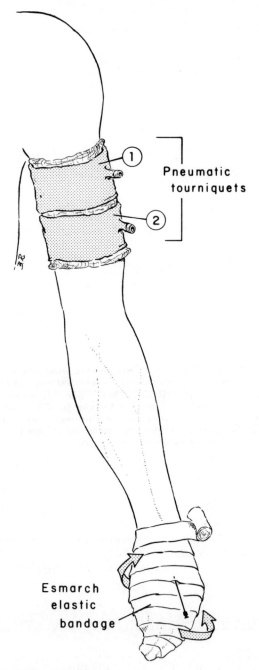

Pneumatic
tourniquets

Esmarch
elastic
bandage

Figure 2-7. Legend on facing page.

tourniquet. This technique has been more recently reported by Holmes,[6] Adams, Dealy, and Kenmore,[1] and others. In the technique recommended by Bell, Slater, and Harris,[2] the dose of lidocaine required is diminished by applying the tourniquet twenty minutes before the anesthetic is injected. "A blood pressure cuff is placed above the elbow and inflated to 200 mm Hg. Twenty minutes later 0.5% lidocaine (5 mgm per ml) is injected into any vein distal to the tourniquet, in a dosage of 1.5 mgm per kg of body weight."[2] Others [1,5] advocate 3.0 mgm per kg.

Under these circumstances anesthesia occurs in several minutes. The tourniquet may produce pain in about forty minutes. A second tourniquet applied distal to the first, in the region of anesthesia, allows release of the first tourniquet and prolongation of comfortable tourniquet time.

This method (figure 2−7) is quite certain. The tourniquet time offers some limitation, and release of the tourniquet causes a loss of anesthesia soon after. The blood vessels are not completely empty during dissection, and some blood staining occurs. Slowing of the pulse and some drop in blood pressure with release of the tourniquet was noted by Finsterbush et al.[5] in 30 percent of 564 patients. This anesthetic agent should be used where toxic reaction can be dealt with if it occurs. When the dosage is kept to 1.5 mgm per kg body weight, toxic reactions have been minimal.

Liver disease and myasthenia are contraindications.

Bibliography

1. Adams, John P.; Dealy, E. J.; and Kenmore, Peter I.: Intravenous lidocaine (Xylocaine) for regional anesthesia in selected hand problems, J. Bone Joint Surg. 46-A: 914−15, 1964.
2. Bell, H. Michael; Slater, Eliot M.; and Harris, William H.: Regional anesthesia with intravenous lidocaine, J.A.M.A. 186:

Figure 2−7. Intravenous regional anesthesia.

1. **Insert needle or polythelene catheter into dorsal vein of hand.**
2. **Wrap extremity with Esmarch bandage.**
3. **Inflate tourniquet (1).**
4. **Remove Esmarch bandage.**
5. **Inject 0.5% lidocaine through previously placed needle or catheter (1.5 to 3.0 mgm/kg body wt).**
6. **Inflate tourniquet (2) if procedure lasts more than thirty minutes and release tourniquet (1).**
7. **Release tourniquet (2) slowly at conclusion of procedure and monitor blood pressure.**

544—49, 1963.

3. Bier, August: Ueber einen neuen Weg Localanästhesie an den Gliedmaassen zu erzeugen, Arch. Klin. Chir. 86:1007—16, 1908.

4. Bromage, Philip R.: Local anaesthetic procedures for the arm and hand, Surg. Clin. North Am. 44, no. 4:919—23, August 1964.

5. Finsterbush, Alexander; Stein, Haim; Robin, Gordon C.; Geller, Raul; and Cotev, Shamay: Recent experiences with intravenous regional anesthesia in limbs, J. Trauma 12:81—84, 1972.

6. Holmes, C. McK.: Intravenous regional analgesia: A useful method of producing analgesia of the limbs, Lancet 1:245—47, 1963.

7. Kasdan, Morton L.; Kleinert, Harold E.; Kasdan, Ann P.; and Kutz, Joseph E.: Axillary block anesthesia for surgery of the hand, Plast. Reconstr. Surg. 46:256—61, 1970.

8. Moore, Daniel C.; Bridenbaugh, L. Donald; and Eather, Kenneth F.: Block of the upper extremity, Arch. Surg. 90:68—72, 1965.

9. Price, James H., and White, Chester W., Jr.: Upper extremity anesthesia by a simple block technique, J. Med. Assoc. State Ala. 35:917—21, 1966.

CHAPTER 3

Joint Stiffness in the Hand

ABSTRACT

The small joints of the hand are very prone to stiffen when held at rest for any reason. Motion may be lost completely from immobilization alone. For this reason, immobilization is a calculated risk. Adjacent fractures and wounds to ligaments and joint capsule make the tendency to stiffen more severe. Adhesions of adjacent tissue layers which normally glide during movement may restrict joint movement severely. Joint stiffening can cause more disability than the original injury.

Pitfalls

1. *Unnecessary joint immobilization*
2. *Lack of passive movement to keep joints mobile when tendons are cut*
3. *Too complete or too long immobilization for fractures and joint wounds*

Normal function of the hand requires free movement of the joints. Situations which may cause deleterious effects on joint movement should be recognized in order to minimize their effects.

These situations are usually one of the following:

1. Immobilization (physical or voluntary, because of pain)
2. Fracture
3. Ligament injury
4. Adjacent wound
5. Edema
6. Systemic disease
7. Congenital anomaly

The fifteen small joints of the digits stiffen readily if held at rest for any reason. It is often forgotten that a normal joint will lose its movement completely if held at rest long enough. Fingers function as a group or team, and one stiff finger gets in the way, inhibiting the use of the others. The degree of joint stiffening from immobilization alone varies with age and from person to person; some people are much more prone to develop stiffness than others, but this is difficult to recognize, which increases the hazard. The young tend to have some protection, but most adults develop significant stiffen-

53

ing in two weeks which becomes permanent if this immobilization interval is extended beyond three or four weeks. Vigorous efforts must be made to restore the full range of movement at the earliest possible time. The longer the period of immobilization, the more difficult is the task of remobilizing the involved joint. It is still not widely recognized that the constant stimulus of movement is required to keep a joint healthy. The nourishment of articular cartilage, the pliability of capsule and collateral ligaments, and other factors all depend on this movement.

The effect of fractures entering the joint with actual disruption of articular surface, causing hemorrhage into or tearing of the joint capsule, is more readily appreciated as a cause of joint stiffness than immobilization alone. The same can be said of ligamentous injury, which may also leave the joint unstable if not repaired early. A wound adjacent to a joint may also limit joint movement because of pain and swelling. Systemic disease (the outstanding example of which is rheumatoid arthritis) and congenital anomalies (failures of development) must be included in the list of etiological factors of joint stiffness. Figure 3–1 is an example of what *not* to allow following a serious hand injury. Immediate extensive cleansing and pedicle grafting could have prevented most of this deterioration.

TISSUE CHANGES WHICH CAUSE JOINT STIFFNESS

Loss of movement may occur from physical changes in the joint itself or its adjacent structures. These may be classified as follows:

1. Changes in joint proper
    a. Alterations of articular surface:
        fracture
        dislocation
        arthritis
    b. Synovial changes:
        adhesions
        changes in synovial fluid
    c. Alterations of capsule and collateral ligaments:
        loss of elasticity
        shortening
        remodeling
2. Changes outside of joint
    a. Adjacent cicatrix
    b. Checkreined tendons
    c. Muscle contractures

It is easy to understand how physical alterations of joint surface can block movement following fractures or arthritic changes. These are readily seen on the x-ray film. Synovial changes are less easily recognized. Evans et al.[4] have shown that the synovial space in the immobilized knee joint of

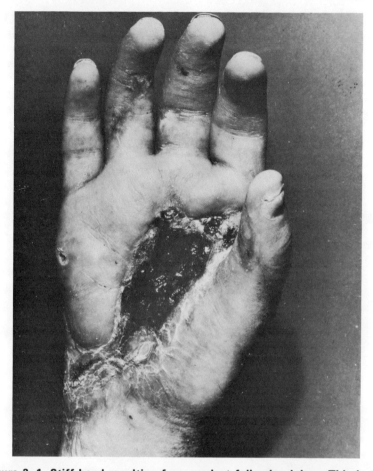

Figure 3–1. Stiff hand resulting from neglect following injury. This is the right hand of a twenty-one-year-old man who caught his hand in the rolls of a machine while at work two months earlier. A large palmar flap of skin became necrotic and the wound was allowed to granulate rather than being covered with a pedicle. Valuable time was lost. The joints were not moved because of swelling, edema, and pain, and they have become irrevocably damaged. Early cleansing and closure with a pedicle could have prevented this.

a rat developed fatty connective tissue which enveloped the cruciate ligaments and the intercondylar notch. This proliferation occurred at fifteen days and was well established by thirty days. The synovial cleft became obliterated, and on remobilization a new cleft for the joint space was formed.

From personal clinical experience with the operative treatment of stiff finger joints and from the work of Akeson,[1] Peacock,[5, 6] and others, I believe that capsule and collateral ligament changes are of the greatest significance in joint stiffening from immobilization. The capsule and collateral ligaments of a joint which has been held at rest for a prolonged period are found to be shorter, thicker, and less pliable than normal. Akeson found a diminution in water and hexosamine content of these tissues. Peacock considers the changes are caused by new collagen formation; Akeson places more emphasis on crossbanding, which occurs in old collagen, as the cause. Whatever the cause, the capsules shorten, become less pliable, and the adjacent

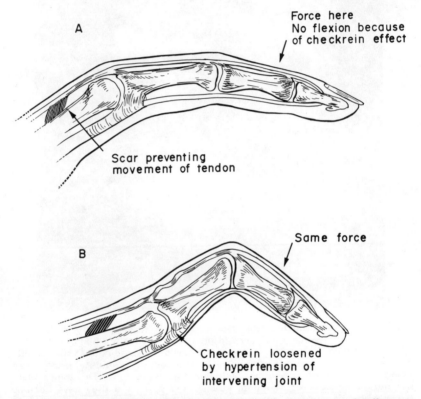

Figure 3–2. *A* Checkrein effect from adherent tendon proximally acts like the checkrein of a horse bridle *B*, can be identified, as shown here, if an intervening joint is used to loosen the involved tendon.

layers of tissue which normally glide over one another become adherent. This is the basis for the surgical intervention in stiff joints advocated by Curtis[3] and for a method of prophylaxis of joint stiffening which will be discussed later in this chapter.

When changes outside the joint interfere with movement, any

alteration in pliability of adjacent tissue will have an adverse effect. This is most striking for scarring secondary to wounds in the vicinity of a joint. It is particularly bad when skin and subcutaneous tissues have healed with the production of a single scar which binds together and prevents differential gliding of the various layers.

Tendons bound in a scar near a joint are very difficult to differentiate from actual joint stiffness. If this "checkrein" is proximal to a second intervening joint, the latter can be placed in an extreme of motion to relax the tendon. When this is done, the first joint is more free to move if it has not stiffened. Relaxing the checkrein does away with its restraining influence (figure 3–2). If both flexor and extensor tendons are checkreined by scar, the test for free movement is not possible. Secondary joint stiffening sets in very rapidly when a joint is held immobile by a checkreined tendon. Also, the process which caused the tendon to become adherent in the first place may well have produced stiffening in the joint. The two conditions frequently exist simultaneously.

Muscle contractures may cause severe alterations in joint movement. The muscle tendon unit is normally pliable, shortening on contraction and expanding on relaxation as the opposing movement-forces operate. If a muscle is partially destroyed so that a large portion of it is replaced by scar, it will no longer be able to lengthen in a normal way and the joint on which it operates will have limited movement. Volkmann's ischemic contracture is the hideous example of this (figure 3–3).

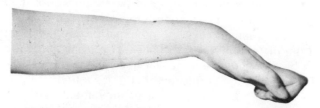

Figure 3–3. Volkmann's contracture of the muscles of the forearm. A ten-year-old girl fell from her bicycle fifteen months earlier, sustaining a fracture of both bones of the left forearm in two areas. The first treatment was by cast, but this was replaced by traction because of extreme swelling of the forearm. The fascia of the forearm was not incised surgically. She lost sensation in her hand as a result of ischemia of the median and ulnar nerves. The muscles of her forearm turned to scar tissue which held her fingers and wrist in flexion because of their contracted pull. This serious complication can be prevented only by restoring circulation to the muscles and nerves of the forearm within hours after the onset. Not only must all constricting casts be removed, but the skin and deep fascia must be incised in most cases to release the pressure.

PREVENTION

Prevention is by far the best approach to the problem of joint stiffness (see figure 3–4). Many physicians do not fully realize that immobilization has both good and bad effects. The problem is to use immobilization cautiously. Bone, tendon, ligament, and, to a lesser extent, nearly every other soft tissue heals more readily in the early stages of repair following injury if it is held at rest. Rest also prevents pain. Because of this, many patients—especially those with a low pain threshold—hold their hand joints at rest. Serious joint stiffening occurs if this continues for any length of time. While an injured tissue which normally transmits force (such as a bone or tendon) must be relieved of this function until its strength is regained, the adverse changes begin as soon as a joint is not moved; these changes rapidly become significant. Joints do not tolerate immobility. They were made for movement. It is unfortunately very common for final disability to be greater from stiffened adjacent joints unwisely held at rest than from an original injury.

If joint immobilization is thought of as a calculated risk, it will properly be kept at a minimum.

1. Do not immobilize unnecessarily.
2. Do not immobilize completely if not necessary.
3. Do not immobilize longer than necessary.
4. Immobilize in position of function when possible.

Leave as many adjacent joints as possible free to move. This is a matter of judgment. Sometimes adjacent joints must be included, but do this with full understanding of the dangers. In the palm, a frequent error is to carry a wrist splint past the level of the *proximal* palmar crease. When this is done, movement of the M-P joints of the fingers is restricted, since the proximal phalanges of the fingers make up the distal quarter of the palm. If a small amount of movement can be allowed, the joint will not stiffen as greatly as if held rigidly. Take advantage of this factor and use it frequently, especially following tendon repair. The range of movement can be restricted without complete fixation of the joint. I prefer cast or splint fixation for joint immobilization rather than Kirschner wire fixation, in most instances, for this same reason. Kirschner wire fixation usually causes more stiffness. The length of immobilization must be judged individually for each situation. In deciding this, the reason for the immobilization should be kept in mind. If it is for relief of pain, more than a few days should not be necessary. If it is to relieve tension on a divided tendon, several weeks may be necessary until continuity of the tendon is reestablished with the strength to transmit the force

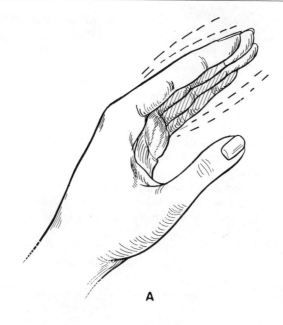

A

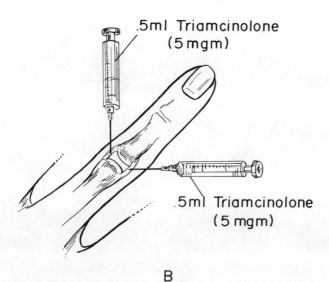

.5ml Triamcinolone
(5 mgm)

.5ml Triamcinolone
(5 mgm)

B

Figure 3–4. Prevention of joint stiffness. *A*, continued joint movement is recommended. *B*, injection of 5 mgm triamcinolone into each collateral ligament is beneficial when mobility is not possible.

to which it is subjected. However, restriction of range of movement without complete immobilization can often be utilized to allow movement in the relaxed position. This restricts the force transmitted through the tendon and, at the same time, is less damaging to the joint.

The position of function (figure 3–5) is the position of balance of the hand. Note that when you hold your own hand in this position it is comfortable. The extensors and flexors are in balance and the thumb is abducted from the index finger. This position is not only comfortable but useful. A flicker of movement allows the thumb to oppose the index fingertip and to provide prehension. When the patient has regained prehension after a period of immobility, he will use his hand, and this in turn leads to more mobility. The position of function is the ideal position which should be used whenever suitable.

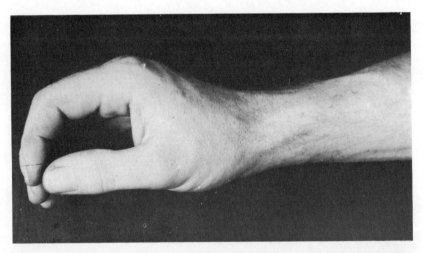

Figure 3–5. Position of function. This is a comfortable position because the flexors and extensors are in balance with the wrist slightly dorsiflexed and the fingers in midflexion. The long axis of the thumb is in line with the shaft of the radius and the thumb tip is adjacent to the tips of the index and long fingers. A flicker of movement gives prehension which, in turn, leads to further use of the hand.

PROPHYLAXIS OF JOINT STIFFNESS WITH TRIAMCINOLONE ACETONIDE

Many situations in elective surgery on the digits of the hand and in the treatment of injuries of the fingers and thumb require immobilization for healing to occur. The idea of a locally injected corticosteroid substance such as triamcinolone seems logical, as it can prevent thickening and tightening of the joint capsule and collateral ligaments of an immobilized joint. When this occurred to me several years ago, I wondered if such injections would prevent or lessen joint stiffening of immobilization. The following experimental work was carried out:

The work of Clark and Weckesser[2] on rats indicates that triamcinolone inhibits or prevents the development of stiffness in the knee joint of a rat which has been held in a fixed position for three weeks by subcutaneous wiring.

Twenty control rats had one knee immobilized in flexion for three weeks by means of a subcutaneous wire and hollow tube. Five of these were given 0.05 ml normal saline intra-articularly into the immobilized knee joint, while the remainder, also immobilized, were not treated in the joint space.

Twenty experimental rats were given 0.5 mgm (2 mgm/kg) triamcinolone acetonide intra-articularly into the immobilized knee joint and six others were given this same dosage into the periarticular ligaments and capsule of the knee joint.

At the end of the three-week period of immobilization, the splinted hind limb was disarticulated at the acetabulum and all soft tissue carefully removed. The femur was then affixed to an adjustable suspending arm as shown in figure 3–6A. The initial angle between the femur and tibia was recorded; then the restraining wire between the tibia and femur was cut and further measurements made. One-half gram weights were added (figure 3–6B). Measurements of the angle were made after the addition of each weight until the joint extended to 100° or until ten grams had been added. One-half of the joints from the experimental animals extended beyond 100° with no weights added to the leg. This happened in none of the control rats (figure 3–6C and D).

The mean weight required to extend the joints of the control animals was 7.5 g, while that of the experimental group was 1.5 g.

Applying this treatment to human patients has been gratifying to date. Immobilization of a finger for thenar pedicle flap replacement of the tip formerly led to rather severe joint stiffness in the finger, but this has been successfully thwarted in twelve patients in which the periarticular tissues of the middle finger joint were infiltrated with triamcinolone acetonide at the time of immobilization.

In view of these experiences, it is now my custom to infiltrate the collateral ligaments and joint capsule of the p.i.p. joint of any adult

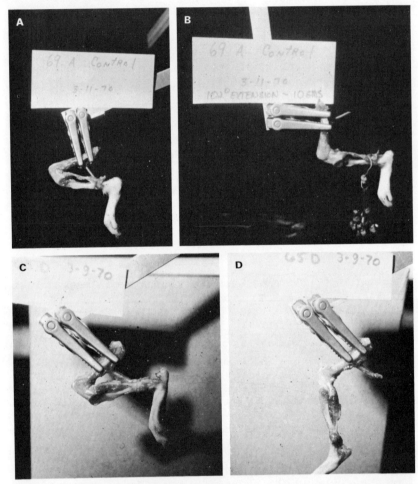

Figure 3–6. Use of triamcinolene to inhibit or prevent stiffness. *A*, the leg of a control rat in the measuring device before cutting the restraining wire between femur and tibia, which had been in place subcutaneously for three weeks. *B*, ten grams of weight were necessary to make the joint of the animal in *A* extend beyond 100°. *C*, the joint of an animal which had 0.5 mgm triamcinolone injected into the periarticular tissues at the time of immobilization three weeks before. The restraining wire is still intact. *D*, extension of the knee joint of the animal in *C* which occurred spontaneously when the wire was cut. No weights have been added.

helpful, but prophylaxis is best.

A power-driven exercise splint, still in the experimental stage, may also prove to be helpful.

Bibliography

1. Akeson, Wayne H.: An experimental study of joint stiffness, J. Bone Joint Surg. 43-A:1022–34, 1961.
2. Clark, D. Dick, and Weckesser, Elden C.: The influence of triamcinolone acetonide on joint stiffness in the rat, J. Bone Joint Surg. 53-A:1409–14, 1971.
3. Curtis, Raymond M.: Joints of the hand, in Flynn, J. Edward (ed.): *Hand Surgery*, pp. 350–76 (Baltimore: Williams & Wilkins Co., 1966).
4. Evans, E. Burke; Eggers, G. W. N.; Butler, James K.; and Blumel, Johanna: Experimental immobilization and remobilization of rat knee joints, J. Bone Joint Surg. 42-A:737–58, 1960.
5. Peacock, Erle E., Jr.: Some biochemical and biophysical aspects of joint stiffness: Role of collagen synthesis as opposed to altered molecular bonding, Ann. Surg. 164:1–12, 1966.
6. Peacock, Erle E., Jr., and VanWinkle, Walton, Jr.: *Surgery and Biology of Wound Repair* (Philadelphia: W. B. Saunders Co., 1970).

CHAPTER 4

Injury to Skin and Subcutaneous Tissue

ABSTRACT

The loss of the normal protective functions of the skin, with puncture wounds, lacerations, and skin avulsions particularly, creates a hazard of infection and fibrosis. These changes may seriously interfere with the function of the moving sensitive parts of the hand.

The wounds should be cleansed and carefully debrided. A head loupe with a magnification of two diameters is helpful. Closure should be carried out at the earliest possible time, usually, to restore the protective function of the skin. If it is necessary to delay treatment for any reason for twelve to twenty-four hours, local antibiotic solution should be applied to the wound after cleansing and systemic antibiotics should be given (delayed emergency). These delayed emergencies are determined on the basis of the condition of the wound, the general condition of the patient, or lack of available personnel. Delay of several days may be necessary in badly contaminated or traumatized wounds. Multiple debridement may be necessary before secondary closure is carried out.

The methods of skin repair are direct suture, local flap rotation, free skin grafting, and pedicle flap coverage from an adjacent or distant area.

Free grafting is suitable if pliable soft tissues remain on which to place the graft. Rotation and pedicle flaps are necessary to supply subcutaneous fat over joints and tendons.

Corticosteroids, such as triamcinolone acetonide, by judicious prophylactic injection into the collateral ligaments and joint capsule can be used to prevent joint stiffness. This is especially useful about the p.i.p. joint in thenar pedicle flaps in older people.

Pitfalls

1. *Retention of foreign bodies in the wound*
2. *Infection because of inadequate cleansing or too early closure*
3. *Unrecognized fracture; tendon or nerve injury*
4. *Unrecognized necrosis of a skin flap in postoperative period*
5. *Hematoma beneath free skin graft*
6. *Joint stiffness because of unnecessary immobilization*

7. *Tight bandage or cast which constricts*
8. *Tetanus or gas gangrene*

Conditions Which Require Very Special Treatment

1. *Loss of skin from an entire digit or a broad area*
2. *Large skin flaps with their base located distally*
3. *Compound injury to bone, tendon, or nerve*
4. *Extreme contamination*

Damage or destruction of skin over any large area of the body is a serious injury. Any penetration or laceration, especially about the hand, can lead to serious consequences. Removal of the protective barrier between the interior of the body and its environment allows fluid and electrolytes to escape and opens the door for invading organisms from the outside. In addition, many delicate structures in the subcutaneous area are laid open to all sorts of adverse influences. The delicate gliding surfaces of the tendons and the synovial surfaces of the many small joints in the area as well as the elastic ligaments which allow joint movement are particularly vulnerable to direct injury, drying, and fibrosis, in addition to infection. This vulnerability of deep structures places a responsibility on the surgeon to restore protection at the earliest time, before irreversible changes take place.

The normal skin and subcutaneous tissues about the dorsum of the hand are very pliable, allowing the movement of the tendons and the fifteen small joints of the digits which makes the part manipulative and prehensile. This pliability must be restored to preserve these functions.

In addition to penetration and laceration, skin may be ground away by abrasion or torn away by finger rings and all sorts of machines with rollers, jaws, and other moving parts. Such machines may avulse or strip away the skin over a broad area. Usually the separation occurs in the loose areolar subcutaneous layer.

Other mechanisms of skin destruction are heat, cold, electricity, and, less frequently, chemicals. Whether the skin is torn away, abraded, or destroyed by extremes of temperature or chemicals, the deeper structures are placed in jeopardy and the route is opened to further injury and bacterial invasion.

Procedures to follow in the treatment of destructive wounds of the hand are:

1. Primary wound closure

    Favorable cases seen early after injury

    a. Wound is cleansed, debrided, irrigated with saline.
    b. Closure of the wound is carried out by:

direct suture
free split thickness skin graft
free full thickness skin graft
rotation skin flap
sliding subcutaneous pedicle flap
primary pedicle flap from near or remote area

2. Delayed primary wound closure—delayed emergency

For wounds suitable for primary closure which, because of special circumstances—usually not related to the wound—must be delayed

   a. After the wound is cleansed, debrided, and irrigated with sterile saline, it is covered with antibiotic locally, and systemic antibiotics are given.
   b. Closure as in 1 can take place up to twenty-four hours later.

3. Secondary wound closure

For less favorable cases in which closure is delayed because of conditions in the wound itself: highly contaminated wounds, blast injuries, high-velocity gunshot wounds, and wounds seen late after injury

   a. Wound is cleansed, irrigated, debrided, but left open.
   b. Two to five days later, closure as in 1. Antibiotics should be given locally and systemically during the interval before closure.
   c. When conditions are quite adverse, multiple debridement may be necessary, as indicated. Minimal immobilization is used postoperatively to avoid unnecessary joint stiffness.

PRIMARY WOUND CLOSURE

Primary wound closure is most desirable and should be utilized when feasible if the contamination is not severe and the case is suitable and seen early. It restores the protection of intact skin at the earliest possible time by the techniques listed on page 67.

DELAYED PRIMARY CLOSURE
(DELAYED EMERGENCY)

Delay in primary closure of a wound, delayed emergency, may be wise because of conditions in the wound itself or because of certain conditions which exist (see chapter 1, page 23). A child with a full stomach who cannot tolerate local anesthesia, a patient with other life-threatening situations which take priority, or, sometimes, the lack of suitable personnel are reasons for delay that fall into this category.

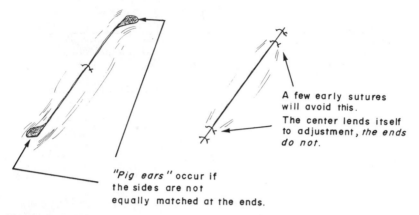

"Pig ears" occur if
the sides are not
equally matched at the ends.

A few early sutures
will avoid this.
The center lends itself
to adjustment, *the ends
do not.*

Figure 4–1. Wound closure by matching the sides of a wound. The best way is to start at the ends.

The skin about the wound should be cleansed with mild detergents, foreign bodies should be removed, and the wound debrided and irrigated as early as possible to diminish the bacterial flora. Local infiltration anesthesia is desirable. Antibiotic solution should be applied in the wound after the primary cleansing, and systemic antibiotics should also be given. One-half percent neomycin solution, 0.1% chloramphenicol, or bacitracin 250–1000 units per ml are examples of antibiotics which can be applied to the wound locally when delay is necessary. With this precaution, the primary closure can be delayed twelve to twenty-four hours until the patient can safely be given a general anesthetic or until other pending situations are corrected. The procedure may need to be altered to fit the particular circumstance.

In less contaminated wounds, delayed primary closure may be utilized because of the condition of the wound. This type of wound is left open for twelve to twenty-four hours before closure is carried out. During this period, local and systemic antibiotics are employed. The protection of immediately restored skin closure is forgone in order to allow adequate inspection and possible drainage. Debridement can be carried out during this period, if necessary. Usually though, when successive debridements are necessary, the closure is later or "secondary."

SECONDARY WOUND CLOSURE

When devitalization and contamination are extreme, the wound is left open for a longer period of time to avoid the danger of infection. When these types of wounds are closed several days or more later, they are arbitrarily called secondary closures. Wounds which necessitate this type of treatment are highly contaminated wounds, blast injuries, high-velocity missile wounds, or wounds seen late after injury.

The open procedure for extreme cases is safer because organisms are not trapped in the wound, the wound can be inspected, and infection, if it occurs, can drain freely to the exterior. During the interval before closure, debridement can be carried out several times in order to free the wound of devitalized tissue. Electrical wounds are examples of wounds in which the line of demarcation actually changes, because of progressive thrombosis in vessels; successive, small stages of debridement are a wise procedure to save as much tissue as possible.

In the interval that the wound is left open, the use of local antibiotics is advised. The longer time-interval before closure and the possible use of multiple debridement distinguish secondary closures from delayed primary wound closures.

FREE SKIN GRAFTING

When the destruction is too wide to allow side-by-side apposition of a wound with sutures (fig 4–1), skin grafting is indicated. The transfer of a sheet of epithelial cells and dermis from one area of the body to another to cover an open wound is, after primary closure, the next most useful technique.

This technique, now a little more than a century old, was first reported by Reverdin[19] in 1869 in the form of "pinch" grafts "the size of a grain of wheat." The demonstration that skin could be successfully transferred from one part of the body to another after complete severance aroused much interest. The technique was modified by Ollier[18] in 1872 and by Thiersch[21] in 1874 to sheets of skin cut horizontally with a straight razor and laid on the open wound or granulating surface to provide epithelial coverage. The basic principles are still the same today. Improvements in equipment for cutting free partial thickness skin grafts have been made and are very useful, but the free-hand art of cutting skin grafts should not be lost.

The types of free skin grafts and methods of obtaining them are:
1. Full thickness—cut with scalpel
2. Partial thickness—cut with:
    free hand blade
    dermatome (Padgett, Reese, Brown)
Figure 4–2 shows some of the various types of equipment available for cutting free skin grafts. The Padgett and Reese dermatomes have the advantage of cutting more uniform and gauged-thickness grafts, while the Brown electric-powered machine allows grafts of great length but with thickness less well-controlled. Each type of machine has certain advantages, and the operator must make his own choice.

With practice, excellent free skin grafts of various thickness can be cut by the free-hand method. These are especially useful in the treatment of wounds of the hand because of their ready availability without special equipment. Small grafts can be readily cut with a sharp stainless steel razor blade held in a hemostat. These can con-

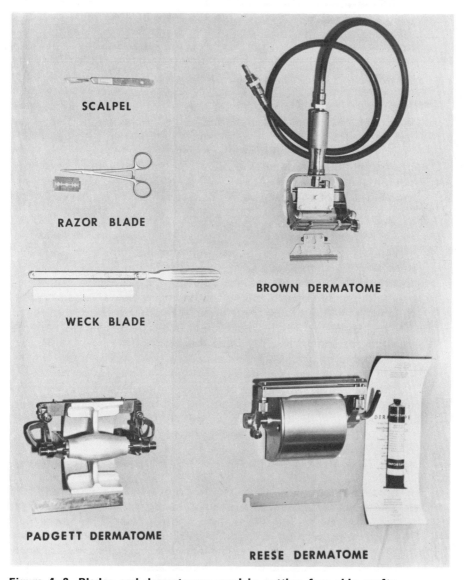

Figure 4–2. Blades and dermatomes used in cutting free skin grafts.

veniently be taken from the forearm. For larger grafts, a broader blade such as the Weck or Blair-Brown is better suited and the thigh donor site produces less visible scarring.

The thicker the graft, the more durable it will be when healed, but the more vulnerable it will be to infection at the time of transfer.

In choosing skin for transfer, it is wise to pick a donor site with texture similar to that which is being replaced, when this is possible. Specialized areas such as the palm, however, have little excess skin for utilization. Lie, Magargle, and Posch[25] utilize full-thickness skin from the hypothenar area. This is fine for small areas such as the fingertip (see chapter 7). The central area of the sole has been advocated, but more often the available areas, such as the inner side of the thigh or the abdominal wall, are utilized, even though the texture of these areas is quite different from the injured portion of the extremity. Transferred epithelium maintains most of the characteristics which it had before transfer. Thigh skin, for example, when placed in the palm, remains quite smooth and glossy and does not provide the same amount of surface traction as the normally grooved skin of the palm. It is a compromise.

Full-Thickness Skin Grafts

Wolfe[24] of Glasgow, an oculist, reported the transfer of full thickness skin (epidermis and dermis) in 1872, and Krause[12] in 1893 reported 100 successful cases of its use.

The donor site usually chosen is the volar surface of the forearm, though it may be any area of the body. A pattern is made of the area to be covered and an enlarged outline of this is made at the donor site to allow for shrinkage. The entire thickness of the skin is removed down to, but not including, the subcutaneous fat. The donor area is closed primarily.

The donor skin with no fat on its deep surface is sutured into place and pressure applied by stent and elastic bandage. Some pressure applied to the graft, up to two weeks after the operation, is helpful in preventing serum accumulation beneath it.

Split-Thickness Skin Grafts

Split-thickness grafts, because they are somewhat more resistant to infection, are most useful on granulating surfaces. Figure 4–3, after May,[15] shows the different thicknesses of split-thickness skin grafts. For granulating wounds, 0.010 to 0.014 inch thickness is most apt to succeed. For replacement of scar, 0.018 to 0.020 inch thickness gives more normal skin texture and is preferred when the graft is placed on a sterile bed where there is little risk of infection.

This gives very good coverage for the back of the hand unless the destruction is very deep, exposing tendons and joints.

Free skin grafting supplies wide epithelial coverage, but does not provide subcutaneous fat and, hence, cannot be applied directly over

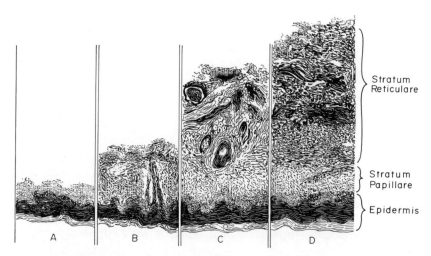

Stratum Reticulare

Stratum Papillare

Epidermis

A　　B　　C　　D

Figure 4–3. Split-thickness skin grafts of various thickness. *A*, very thin, *B*, thin (0.010 inch). *C*, thick partial thickness (0.022 inch). *D*, full thickness. (Reproduced, with permission, from Hans May, *Plastic and Reconstructive Surgery*, 3rd ed. [Philadelphia: F. A. Davis Co., 1971])

moving parts such as joint and tendon. The pliability necessary for the proper functioning of these structures requires the transfer of subcutaneous fat as well as skin.

SHIFTING OF SKIN AND SUBCUTANEOUS TISSUES

The shifting of skin and subcutaneous tissues may be divided into three types:
1. Shifting of adjacent tissues
   a. Undercutting
   b. Rotation
   c. Sliding subcutaneous pedicle flap:
      no skin bridge
      subcutaneous tissue undetached
      nourishment by vessels in subcutaneous pedicle

(as done by Kutler,[13] Barron and Emmett,[2] Trevaskis et al.[22])
2. Pedicle flaps from nearby
    a. Thenar
    b. Cross-finger
    c. Island:
        no skin bridge
        subcutaneous tissue completely detached except vessels and nerves
        nourishment by vessels in subcutaneous pedicle
3. Pedicle flaps from a distance
    a. Immediate:
        open
        closed by skin graft or by tubing
    b. Delayed: closed by skin graft or by tubing
    c. "Crane" principle for subcutaneous transfer

The shifting or transfer of subcutaneous tissue along with skin requires retention of blood supply from the donor site at least until a new blood supply is developed at the recipient area. The simplest form of skin and subcutaneous tissue transfer occurs in the under-cutting and sliding together of the adjacent skin edges of a broad wound.

If, however, by additional incisions a rectangle or other shape of skin and subcutaneous tissue is elevated which receives its blood supply from the remaining skin attachment, it is spoken of as a *skin flap* because if it is attached only at one side or area. This area of attachment, particularly if it is narrow, is also spoken of as a *pedicle* since it is the foot or stem through which the blood supply is carried. If a ribbon of skin and subcutaneous tissue is elevated but remains attached at each end, it is a *bipedicle flap*. If a ribbon of skin of shorter length is elevated and divided so that only one end or side is attached, it is a *single pedicle flap*. If the edges of the ribbon of skin still attached at each end are sewed to each other, a closed tube can be formed which remains sterile. (The donor area must be sutured or covered with a free open graft.) This is called a *tubed pedicle flap* (Filatov,[6] Gillies[10]). If the flap is immediately transferred to a recipient area, it is a *primary pedicle flap*; if it is formed and allowed to heal before transfer, it is called a *secondary* or *delayed pedicle flap*. Primary pedicle flaps should have broader bases than delayed ones.

The operation of partially severing the blood supply of a pedicle flap and restoring the skin back into its original site is spoken of as a *delay*. This operation is used to increase the blood supply by gradually narrowing the base or to increase the blood supply from the recipient bed prior to detachment and thus make the detachment safer.

Pedicle flaps have been devised in many ingenious ways to transfer tissue. Usually there is a skin bridge that is not divided until a new blood supply is established at the recipient area. The blood vessels in the undivided skin and subcutaneous tissue nourish the flap up to the time of detachment. The sliding subcutaneous pedicle flap and the island pedicle flap are exceptions in that they have no bridge of skin.

The sliding subcutaneous pedicle flap receives its blood supply through undivided subcutaneous tissue (Kutler,[13] Barron and Emmett,[2] Trevaskis et al.[22]) It has broad subcutaneous attachment which is stretched as the skin flap is transferred.

The island pedicle flap is transferred with only its vessels and nerve attached, the skin and subcutaneous tissue being completely severed at the first stage except for the pedicle.

Deeper structures may be included in a pedicle flap (*compound flap*), but usually skin and subcutaneous fat are the two main tissues transferred. Millard[16] has advocated the use of the pedicle flap as a "crane" to supply subcutaneous tissue. The pedicle flap is detached, leaving a "blanket" of transferred subcutaneous tissue, and returned to its original donor area at the end of one week. A free skin graft is applied to the transferred "blanket of subcutaneous tissue" five days later. Crockett[4] has utilized the principle with limited success and states that skin-to-skin approximation of the pedicle is not mandatory.

GENERAL PRINCIPLES FOR MAKING PEDICLE FLAPS

1. The pedicle should be of tissue as similar to that which it is to replace as possible.
2. It should be slightly larger to allow for shrinkage.
3. It should have a broad enough base to provide adequate circulation. This varies in different parts of the body with age and especially if a large artery and vein can also be included (for example, in the groin area where the inferior epigastric vessels can be employed, as advocated by Shaw and Payne[20]). If no large vessels can be utilized, the flap should be nearly as wide as it is long. It is safest to keep the pedicle less than one and one-half times longer than it is wide. Any shorter length than this gives even greater safety. A nearly square pedicle is safest. Experience and judgment are required to elevate pedicles of significant size without going beyond the critical limits of circulatory safety. When in doubt, it is better to replace the flap and make the elevation in successive stages so that nature can increase the circulation before the transfer is made.
4. In addition to having proper size and consistency and adequate

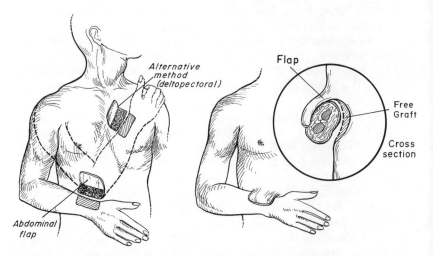

Figure 4–4. Direct flap graft. For defects requiring skin and subcutaneous tissue on the margin of the forearm or hand, the direct flap is best suited. The donor area is covered with a free partial-thickness skin graft. The abdomen or the deltopectoral area may be used.

circulation, the tissue should be transferred without infection to prevent fibrosis. This is done by maintaining skin coverage over the subcutaneous tissues at all times. It is accomplished by direct closure, free grafting of the undersurface of the flap, or by tubing. Each of these methods has its place, and frequently a combination of techniques is employed.

Free grafting of the donor area and undersurface is most applicable to primary direct flaps, as shown in figure 4–4. A free skin graft to the donor area can be carried up on the undersurface of the pedicle flap to the nearest margin of the recipient wound in order to give complete closure. Pressure is then applied to the graft by suturing a stent of fluff, gauze, cotton, or other soft material over the graft.

Tubing of a ribbon of pedicle tissue in order to maintain skin coverage and to maintain a closed surface was first reported by Filatov[6] in 1917 and popularized by Gillies[10] of London soon after. It is particularly suited for longer pedicles which can be utilized to cover defects not accessible at the margins of an extremity.

5. The amount of contact of the pedicle to the recipient area should be as great as possible at the first stage. This ensures a broad base new vascular attachment and makes subsequent steps safer by increasing the new blood supply. Since these pedicles are longer, they must be prepared beforehand, usually in stages, so that sufficient blood supply is developed through one end of the tube, which is left attached at the donor area while the other end is carried to the recipient defect. By multiple "delay" stages a rather

large flat area of tissue can be vascularized and carried on the free end of the tube, if desired (as shown in figure 4–5), or the end of the tube itself may be opened partially and applied to the recipient area. The tube pedicle allows application to less accessible areas because of its greater length and greater freedom of rotation. It requires greater time for preparation, which is a drawback; at present it is utilized only when a primary pedicle flap is not feasible.

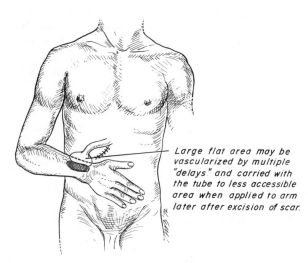

Large flat area may be vascularized by multiple "delays" and carried with the tube to less accessible area when applied to arm later after excision of scar.

Figure 4–5. Tube pedicle flap graft. The tubed pedicle flap being longer than the direct flap allows application to less accessible areas away from the margin of the extremity. A ribbon of skin and subcutaneous tissue is raised and sutured into a tube by a suture line on its undersurface. The donor area is either skin grafted or closed directly with sutures, as shown here. The end of this "tubed" pedicle is freed and transferred to a recipient area, usually at a later stage. If the tube is transferred primarily, it must be quite short.

DELTOPECTORAL PEDICLE FLAP

A pedicle flap from the upper chest wall has been developed for pharyngo-esophageal reconstruction by Bakamjian.[26] The tip of this flap is taken from the acromial or subacromial region, with the base located medially to include the perforating branches of the internal mammary artery from interspaces two, three, or four. This has been adapted to use in hand reconstruction by Stein and Morgan.[27] It has a good arterial blood supply, can be tubed acutely, and has dependent drainage for the pedicle and also for the hand (see figure 4–4).

THENAR PEDICLE FLAP

A number of special types of pedicles are useful about the hand. Figure 4–6 shows the use of a flap of the thenar eminence skin and subcutaneous tissue to close the end of an amputated finger (see chapter 8). Thenar skin has the advantage of being similar to fingertip skin. By elevating the thenar flap transversely, as originally done by Gatewood,[8] it can be made to cover the volar portion of the distal pad of the finger also. The finger, in being sutured in rather acute flexion for the three-week period required for transfer, may become quite stiffened in its interphalangeal joints, however. This is a distinct disadvantage, especially for older people whose joints stiffen more

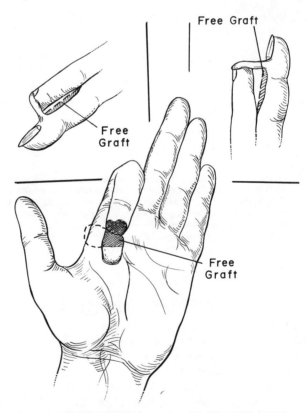

Free Graft

Free Graft

Free Graft

Figure 4–6. Thenar pedicle flap graft. The thenar pedicle flap can be used to replace fingertip tissue when necessary. Joint stiffening of the middle joint of the finger can be prevented by the periarticular injection of a small amount (1/2 ml) of corticosteroid, such as triamcinolone acetonide, into each collateral ligament prophylactically.

readily. It can now be prevented by periarticular injection of corticosteroid, such as 1/2 ml (5 mgm) of triamcinolone acetonide, into each collateral ligament of the p.i.p. joint. The donor thenar area is covered with a free full-thickness or split-thickness skin graft in the first stage. This grafted area at the base of the thumb is sometimes considered a disadvantage because of noticeable scarring or sensitivity, although it usually causes no disability. Hypothenar skin works well here.

CROSS-FINGER PEDICLE FLAP

Tissue from an adjacent digit used to cover a defect, a cross-finger pedicle flap, is shown in figure 4–7; this has the advantage of ready availability and requires no immobilization beyond the injured hand, making for limited disability during convalescence. This technique has been widely used since reported by Gurdin and Pangman.[11]

However, dorsal skin is usually utilized for volar defects. Complete

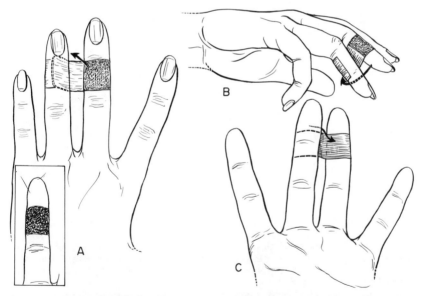

Figure 4–7. Cross-finger flap graft. This illustration shows a flap from the dorsum of the long finger used to cover the volar surface of the ring finger. The cross-finger pedicle flap allows the transfer of tissue from one digit to another. The donor area is covered with a free skin graft. (See also figure 10-3B).

detachment during the two stages of transfer requires nerve regrowth into the transferred tissue and, as a result, reduces sensitivity in the transferred tissue. On rare occasions some disability occurs with the donor digit. Prophylactic periarticular corticosteroid injection is recommended about the p.i.p. joint, although the tendency to stiffen is less than with the thenar flap.

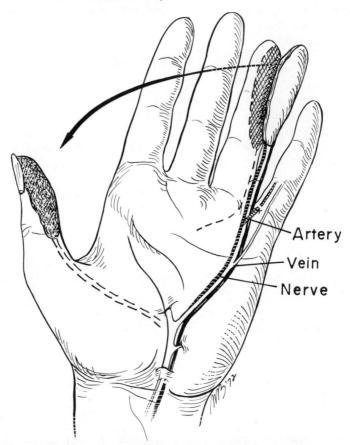

Figure 4–8. Island pedicle flap graft. The island pedicle flap provides replacement of subcutaneous tissue and skin with normal sensation to an area within reach of the vessels and nerve of the donor island. The vessels and nerve are carefully dissected free to maintain circulation and sensation during the transfer, which is made at one stage. It is particularly suited for the restoration of tissue with normal sensation to the radial part of the hand. The donor area is covered with a free graft and has limited sensation. The vessels and nerve are either tunneled subcutaneously to their new location or transferred there through open incision. When using this technique or the cross-finger flap technique care must be taken to prevent kinking or pressure.

ISLAND PEDICLE FLAP

The island pedicle flap uses a remarkable and unique method of tissue transfer (shown in figure 4—8) which has much in its favor for use about the hand where sensation is so very important. The nerve and blood supply of the transferred tissue remain uninterrupted from the moment of transfer. Credit for the development of this operation belongs to Gersuny,[9] Esser,[5] Bunnell,[3] Littler,[14] Moberg,[17] Tubiana and Duparc,[23] Frackelton and Teasley,[7] and others.

The skin is completely divided at the very first stage, producing the "island" which remains attached to its neurovascular bundle. Because of this, it is well suited to bring normal sensation into an important area of opposition, such as the opposing surfaces of the thumb or index finger. It can also be utilized to bring added blood supply to an ischemic digit.

The advantages of the island pedicle are normal sensation and increased blood supply to the recipient area. The disadvantages of the operation are:

1. Limited length of the neurovascular pedicle
2. Sacrifice of normal sensation on the donor area
3. Diminution of vascularity of the donor and adjacent border of the adjacent digit
4. Lack of two remaining patent digital arteries in damaged fingers

There are several determining factors in planning the island pedicle flap.

1. It should be determined that the donor finger has two patent digital arteries. The digital Allen test (figure 4—9) can be utilized for this purpose.
2. Utilizing a piece of string or tape, the suitability of the island for transfer should be determined by measuring the length of the neurovascular pedicle to determine whether or not it will reach the new site.
3. A pattern slightly larger than the defect to be replaced should be outlined (if possible) on the side of the donor finger to be utilized. In my opinion, the size of the donor island should not exceed approximately one-half the volar aspect of the distal portion of the finger beyond the midportion of the middle phalanx, although larger islands have been utilized.

Technique for Island Pedicle Flap

After proper anesthesia, skin sterilization, and sterile draping, the blood is drained from the extremity by elevation and wrapping with a

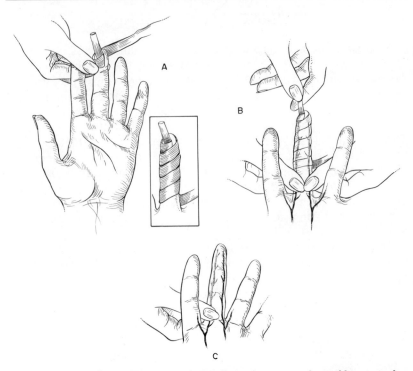

Figure 4−9. The digital Allen test. *A*, the finger is exsanguinated by wrapping with a rubber Penrose drain. *B*, blanching persists if compression is held after removal of the drain. *C*, when compression on a patent artery is released, the finger becomes pink. (Redrawn, with permission, from Ashbell, Kutz, and Kleinert, The digital Allen test, Plastic and Reconstructive Surgery 39:311−12, 1967. Copyright 1967 The Williams & Wilkins Co., Baltimore)

sterile elastic bandage. The pneumatic cuff tourniquet pressure is then inflated to approximately 250 mm Hg.

An outline of the island of skin and subcutaneous tissue to be transferred is made with a marking pen on the side of the distal portion of the donor finger.

A midlateral incision is made on the side of the chosen digit, usually the ulnar side of the ring finger, to the base of the outlined island.

Dissection is carried to the neurovascular bundle which is then gently dissected free from surrounding tissue. An ocular loupe with a magnification of two diameters is very helpful during this stage of the operation.

Dissection of the neurovascular bundle is carried distally to the base of the island. The dorsal branches of the artery and vein must be transected and ligated, leaving the main digital vessels and the digital nerve unimpaired.

After the neurovascular pedicle has been dissected free from the base of the finger to the base of the outlined island of donor skin and elevated with small pieces of rubber tissue clamped in mosquito forceps, the incision is completed about the outline of the island. This must be dissected free from the underlying tendon tunnel, again taking great care not to injure the neurovascular pedicle where it joins the island at its proximal margin. When this has been done, the island and its pedicle can be elevated with a skin hook to the base of the digit. The skin incision should be zigzagged into the palm, following the lines of the skin as much as possible. As the neurovascular pedicle is freed into the palm, the division of the origin of the digital artery to the adjacent digit comes into view. Depending upon the length of the pedicle required for the transfer, it may be necessary to sever the digital artery from the adjacent digit. Usually this will be necessary. After the artery is cut, the neurovascular pedicle can be freed to the level of the midpalmar crease, making the mobilization complete. The tourniquet should be released at this point to test circulation.

In order to move the pedicle to its new location on the thumb or index finger, it is either tunneled there wholly or in part or carried over through additional zigzag incisions of the palm which follow skin lines and creases. It is most important to free the neurovascular pedicle throughout its course. I have no hesitancy in making additional incisions to be certain of this. Circulation is again checked with the island in its new location. The island should quickly return to a healthy pink color with the release of pressure.

The island is then sutured into place at the recipient area, a free thick split-thickness skin graft from the thigh is placed over the donor area, and a pressure stent applied by tying the marginal sutures over it. The balance of the wounds are closed and soft dressings of gauze are applied to all areas, leaving the transferred island readily accessible for inspection of circulation. An elastic bandage is utilized over the grafted donor area, but not over the transferred island or its neurovascular pedicle, which should be left free of pressure.

Z-PLASTY OR N-PLASTY FLAPS

The transposition of triangular flaps from the sides of a wound has many uses. It is, first of all, a method of increasing the length of a wound when excess tissue from the sides is present. The triangular flaps, as shown in figure 4—10, are rotated and shifted to interdigitate in a new, interchanged position. This gives a zigzag shape to the incision instead of a straight line. This can also be very useful when

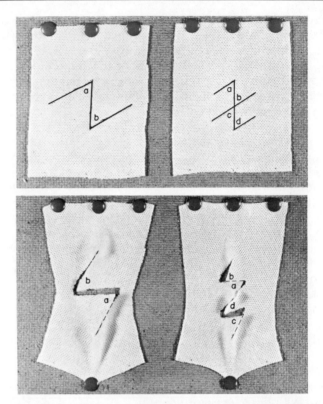

Figure 4–10. Demonstration of Z-Plasty. *A,* **on the left is a single Z with equal limbs of 3 cm each. The side arms make 60° angles with the central limb. On the right are two half-size Zs with the same angles.** *B,* **they have both been lengthened an equal amount. Note that as the length is increased the triangular flaps rotate and shift from side to side to produce narrowing. This narrowing is more broadly distributed with the two small sets of flaps than with the large single set of flaps. Note also that the new transverse arm lies along a line connecting the two original side arms.**

a laceration crosses a normal flexion crease. The crease can be restored by this technique during primary closure. The transverse arm of the zigzag closure will lie in a line connecting the ends of the two side arms.[29] The increase in length thus provided can also be used to make skin conform to irregularities of contour, such as the clefts between the digits.

There are different ways of considering the changes that occur when the flaps are shifted. Limberg[28] points out that the process may be considered as the deformation of a parallelogram by lengthening the short dimension and shortening the long dimension, thus bringing in the tissues from the sides. Another concept is that each triangular flap, as it crosses to the opposite side, acts as a wedge to produce lengthening of that side. In each instance, tissues are brought in from the sides to make the wound longer.

Many interesting relationships exist regarding the angle between the vertical wound and the side arms and between the length of the side arms. The greater the angle between the central wound and the side arm, the greater the effect. Of course, the larger the triangular flaps, the greater the effect.

Figure 4–10B demonstrates that two small sets of triangular flaps distribute the narrowing over a broader area than a single large set of triangular flaps.

Sixty-degree angles between the central wound and the side arms give flaps which are effective and yet not too narrow for adequate circulation.

There are many variables. For practical purposes remember the following:

1. The tissues must be lax from side to side in order to exchange the triangular flaps.
2. If sufficient lateral laxity is not present, the flaps will not interchange.
3. Narrowing will occur equal to the lengthening which is accomplished.
4. Angles of 60° make good triangular flaps.
5. The two bilateral arms are best made parallel to each other. (This means that the two angles are made equal.)
6. The new transverse line will lie in a line connecting the ends of the two side arms. (For 60° angles and side arms equal to the length of the center wound, this will be transverse.)[29]
7. Lengthening is proportional to the size of the Z-plasty.
8. Lengthening is proportional to the size of the angle from the center wound. (The difficulty of exchanging the flaps also increases.)
9. For 60° angles and side arms and center arm of equal length, the lengthening will be 73 percent.
10. Two or more small Z-plasties distribute the narrowing over a broader area than a single large Z-plasty.

Y-V ADVANCEMENT

A single triangular flap can be advanced from one side to lengthen a tight area of skin. A primary incision in the shape of a Y is made transverse to the area of tightness. The flap is advanced across the tight area as it is closed in a V shape (figure 4–11).

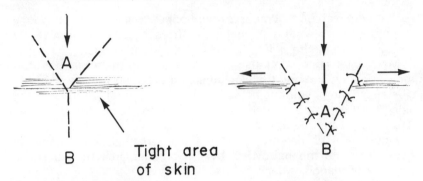

B   Tight area   B
of skin

Figure 4–11. Y-V advancement. Incise as a Y and close as a V across an area of tightness. Note that in this instance the design is transverse in contrast to the central limb of the Z in the Z-plasty, which is parallel with the tight area which is to be lengthened.

Bibliography

1. Ashbell, T. Shelly; Kutz, Joseph E.; and Kleinert, Harold E.: The digital Allen test, Plast. Reconstr. Surg. 39:311–12, 1967.
2. Barron, J. N., and Emmett, A. J. J.: Subcutaneous pedicle flaps, Br. J. Plast. Surg. 18:51–78, 1965.
3. Bunnell, Sterling: Digit transfer by neurovascular pedicle, J. Bone Joint Surg. 34-A:772–74, 1952.
4. Crockett, David J.: The Millard "crane flap" for acute hand injuries, Hand 2:156–59, 1970.
5. Esser, J. F. S.: Island flaps, N.Y. State J. Med. 106:264–65, 1917.
6. Filatov, V. P.: Plastic procedure using a round pedicle (trans. Labunka, Miroslav; Gnudi, Martha Teach; and Webster, Jerome P., from Vestn. Oftalmol. 34, nos. 4–5: 149–58, 1917), Surg. Clin. North Am. 39, no. 2:277–87, April 1959.
7. Frackelton, William H., and Teasley, Jack L.: Neurovascular island pedicle—extension in usage, J. Bone Joint Surg. 44-A: 1069–72, 1962.
8. Gatewood, M. D.: A plastic repair of finger defects without hospitalization, J.A.M.A. 87:1479, 1926.
9. Gersuny, Rob.: Plastischer Ersatz der Wangenschleimhaut, Zentralbl. Chir. 14:706–8, 1887.
10. Gillies, H. D.: The tubed pedicle in plastic surgery, N.Y. State J. Med. 111:1–4, 1920.
11. Gurdin, Michael, and Pangman, W. John: The repair of surface defects of fingers by transdigital flaps, Plast. Reconstr. Surg. 5:368–71, 1950.

12. Krause, Fedor: Ueber die transplantation grosser ungestielter Hautlappen, Verh. Dtsch. Ges. Chir. 22, pt. 2:46, 1893.
13. Kutler, William: A new method for finger tip amputation, J.A.M.A. 133:29–30, 1947.
14. Littler, J. William: Neurovascular pedical transfer of tissue in reconstructive surgery of the hand, J. Bone Joint Surg. 38-A: 917, 1956.
15. May, Hans: *Plastic and Reconstructive Surgery* 3rd ed., p. 26 (Philadelphia: F. A. Davis Co., 1971).
16. Millard, D. Ralph: The crane principle for the transport of subcutaneous tissue, Plast. Reconstr. Surg. 43:451–62, 1969.
17. Moberg, Eric: Discussion of Donal Brooks: The place of nerve-grafting in orthopaedic surgery, J. Bone Joint Surg. 37-A: 305, 326, 1955.
18. Ollier, L.: Les greffes cutanées ou autoplastiques, Bull. Acad. Méd. 1, 2d ser., 243–50, 1872.
19. Reverdin, J. L.: Greffe épidermique, Bull. Soc. Imp. Chir. Paris 10:493–511, 1869.
20. Shaw, Darrel T., and Payne, Robert L., Jr.: One stage tubed abdominal flaps: Single pedicle tubes, Surg. Gynecol. Obstet. 83:205–9, 1946.
21. Thiersch, C.: Ueber die feineren anatomischen Veränderungen bei Aufheilung von Haut auf Granulationen, Arch. Klin. Chir. Berlin 17:318, 1874.
22. Trevaskis, Allan E.; Rempel, John; Okunski, Walter; and Rea, Michael: Sliding subcutaneous-pedicle flaps to close a circular defect, Plast. Reconstr. Surg. 46:155–57, 1970.
23. Tubiana, R., and Duparc, J.: Restoration of sensibility in the hand by neurovascular skin island transfer, J. Bone Joint Surg. 43-B:474–80, 1961.
24. Wolfe, J.R.: A method of performing plastic operations, Br. Med. J. 2:360, 1875.

FREE FULL-THICKNESS GRAFTS FROM PALM
25. Lie, Kim K.; Magargle, Ronald K.; Posch, Joseph L.: Free full-thickness skin grafts from palm to cover defects of the fingers, J. Bone Joint Surg. 52-A:599–61, 1970.

DELTOPECTORAL PEDICLE FLAP
26. Bakamjian, V. Y.: A two-stage method for pharyngoesophageal reconstruction with a primary pectoral skin flap, Plast. Reconstr. Surg. 36:173–84, 1965.
27. Stein, Frank, and Morgan, L. Richard: The use of the Bakamjian flap in reconstruction of the hand. Paper presented at Twenty-seventh Annual Meeting of The American Society for Surgery of the Hand, 29 January 1972, Washington, D.C.

Z-PLASTY
28. Limberg, Alexander A.: Design of local flaps, in Gibson, Thomas (ed.): *Modern Trends in Plastic Surgery*, 2d ser., pp. 38–61 (London: Butterworth, 1966).
29. McGregor, Ian A.: *Fundamental Techniques of Plastic Surgery and Their Surgical Applications*, 4th ed., p. 6 (Baltimore: Williams & Wilkins Co., 1968).

CHAPTER 5

The Treatment of Burns, Chemical Injury, and Frostbite

ABSTRACT

Although the damage from heat or cold is greatest on the surface, it may extend to deep tissues. The extent of injury is often very difficult, if not impossible, to gauge immediately after injury. Local treatment should emphasize cleansing, periodic exercise of the fingers, and rest on splints in the position of function. The systemic effects of severe burns take priority. Burns involving both upper extremities constitute nearly 20 percent of the body surface and may require intravenous fluids. The urine output should be kept at 30—50 ml per hour. Burns which represent full thickness destruction of skin on the hand may be best treated by primary excision and grafting when the systemic condition of the patient permits; otherwise skin coverage should be restored at the earliest time that the condition of the patient and the wound permit.

Chemical injuries are best treated by neutralization and copious washing. Phosphorus burns—common in warfare because phosphorus is used in smoke screens, incendiary bombs, and tracer bullets—are also best treated by copious washing, removal of the particles, and alkalinization.

Hydrofluoric acid burns should be treated with calcium gluconate injected into the adjacent tissues after copious washing.

Frostbite is best prevented by proper protective clothing. Blanching and numbness are danger signs. Parts should be warmed quickly when this occurs. Rapid thawing in hot water 40° to 42°C (104° to 108°F) is recommended. This is painful and requires medication. After rapid thawing, the part should be kept at a room temperature. Intravenous dextran and anticoagulants as well as sympathetic blocks are of value.

Pitfalls—Burns

   1. Depth of burn greater than anticipated
   2. Systemic effects of burn unrecognized
   3. Shock

4. *Infection*
5. *Joint stiffness*

Pitfalls—Chemical Injury

1. *Failure to wash and neutralize acid or alkali burns*
2. *Failure to remove retained materials from wound*
3. *Failure to utilize calcium gluconate in hydrofluoric acid burns*

Pitfalls—Frostbite

1. *Failure of patient to wear protective clothing*
2. *Failure of patient to heed the warning signs of blanching or numbness*
3. *Failure to thaw part in hot water (104° to 108°F)*
4. *Rubbing the frozen part in snow*
5. *Omission of aids to circulation after thawing*

When the upper extremity is subjected to extremely high temperatures, tissue injury occurs which is greatest at the skin surface but which diminishes as the tissues are penetrated. Hurley, Ham, and Ryan[8] produced a skin burn on rats with capillary and venule damage by applying a copper disk at 54°C (128.4°F) for twenty seconds. Reduction of the temperature to 51°C (123°F) avoided microscopic vascular damage, indicating this temperature as marginal for damage under these conditions. In similar experiments with guinea pigs, there was a 10° difference between the surface temperature applied and that at the deep aspect of the dermis, indicating a very rapid drop in temperature as the tissues are penetrated—if the temperatures are not high above the damage level.

First degree injury involves erythema without actual destruction of tissue cells. Partial thickness or second degree burning produces blistering and partial destruction in which a portion of the deep layers of the epithelium or some cells of the hair follicles and sweat glands of the dermis remain and from which proliferation and epithelialization can occur. Third degree burning implies that all epithelial elements are destroyed. Further grading of injury to include deep subcutaneous damage has been made since the time of Dupuytren, but the usual grading is on the basis of skin injury.

The extent of the injury depends upon the temperature involved, the length of time it is applied, and the presence of clothing or garments which may hold the heat. The thick palmar skin can withstand a higher temperature than that of the back of the hand. The hand, because of its function of grasp, is frequently involved with hot objects.

There are many possible effects on the hand from burns:
1. Skin loss
2. Exposure of deep structures
3. Destruction of deep structures
4. Infection
5. Edema
6. Scarring
7. Joint stiffness

The destruction or serious damage to the skin of the hand by external heat creates a necessity for restoration of skin continuity at the earliest possible time in order to prevent any or all of the adverse effects just listed, as well as to preserve voluntary movement in the many small joints. Proper hand function depends upon the free movement of the joints of each digit. This movement, in turn, requires loose pliable skin which will allow flexion and extension of each joint. The ligaments and capsules of the joints must not be allowed to thicken and fibrose from immobility, infection, or edema during the time that the burn is healing. This is best prevented by daily exercises in a saline or mild detergent bath, at which time the wounds are gently cleansed. After a period of twenty to thirty minutes of exercise in the bath, the bacteriostatic applications are reapplied to the burn areas and the hand is either loosely dressed with soft gauze or left exposed and allowed to rest in the position of function on a sterilized splint of metal or other suitable material. (See figure 3–5, page 60, for the position of function: wrist in dorsiflexion, fingers in midflexion, and thumb in abduction.)

The advantage of the position of function, in addition to holding the hand in its most balanced position, is the facility with which a small amount of movement leads to prehension between the thumb and the index finger.

The management of burns of the hand varies with the size and depth of the burn and the extent of other body surface that is involved. These factors are taken into consideration in the outline of treatment.

The systemic effects of burns must also be considered:
1. Early effects: fluid loss → burn shock
2. Later effects: bacterial invasion → sepsis
Death can result from either of these.

The urine output is an excellent guide to fluid therapy in the early post-burn state. This should be maintained at or about 30 to 50 ml per hour. Systemic antibiotics and tetanus immunization are also in order. Blood transfusions are required to maintain a near normal hemoglobin concentration.

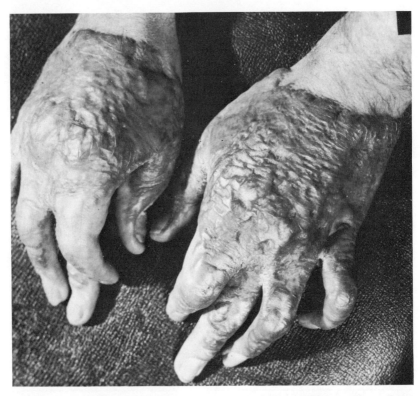

Figure 5–1. Neglected third degree burn in an aviator taken prisoner. Hand movement is almost nil because of the one-and-one-half-centimeter-thick scar of the back of the hand.

For an excellent review of the systemic treatment of burns, the reader is referred to the monograph by Artz and Moncrief[1] and that of Shuck, Moncrief, and Monafo.[15]

When burns of the hand are associated with burns of other parts of the body, the systemic aspects of the injury frequently become most important because the injury is a threat to life. This depends on the depth and the extent of the burn area. Burns of 20 percent of the body surface area require intravenous fluid resuscitation. The surface area of an upper extremity is usually considered about one-half of this amount.

If the exposure is confined to one upper extremity (approximately 9 percent of total body surface), the early systemic effects from fluid loss should not be excessive. However, the danger of infection may be great, and the later crippling effect from scarring may be severe. In burns confined to the hands, the adverse effects are particularly those of scar formation which interferes with the normal movements of the hand (see figure 5–1). To avoid scarring, it is important to prevent infection which destroys the remaining epithelial islands and to apply skin grafts early if all epithelium has been destroyed. Primary excision and closure or skin grafting is indicated when destruction is definitely full-thickness, as shown in figure 5–3A. I favor this treatment, if the area is anesthetic, to diminish impairment of function. If there is question about full-thickness destruction, however, it is better to wait, apply local antibiotics, and reevaluate after the eschar is separated. The delay should be as short as possible.

The use of skin from another individual (homograft) or from an animal (heterograft) as a temporary dressing is a new method with considerable potential which offers a method of sterilizing the burn wound.[2, 12, 13]

PRIMARY LOCAL TREATMENT OF BURNS OF THE HAND

Procedure for local primary treatment of burns (figure 5–2) about the hand is outlined according to the extent of injury.

1. Partial thickness burns, in this order:
   Gentle cleansing with detergent
   Application of local bacteriostatic agent, for example, mafenide acetate (Sulfamylon cream), bacitracin ointment, or polymyxin B-bacitracin-neomycin (Neosporin ointment)
   Cock-up splint for severe cases. (Mild cases can be covered with bacteriostatic agent and soft dressing, without splinting; this allows movement and prevents joint stiffening.)
2. Full thickness burns
   a. Primary excision and immediate skin coverage if burn is circumscribed and the general condition of the patient permits:
      primary closure of wound
      primary skin grafting
      splint in position of function
   b. Delayed skin coverage, in this order:
      gentle cleansing with detergent
      application of bacteriostatic agent
      cock-up sterile splint
      twice daily baths and exercises before reapplying bacteriostatic agent
      debridement (surgical for gross removal of dead tissue; proteolytic enzymes for microscopic removal)

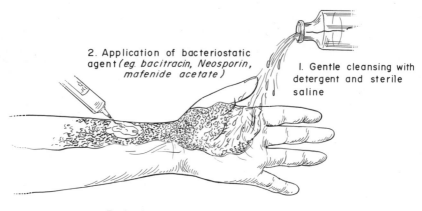

2. Application of bacteriostatic agent *(eg. bacitracin, Neosporin, mafenide acetate)*

1. Gentle cleansing with detergent and sterile saline

3. Cock—up splint for severe cases

4. Periodic exercise to diminish joint stiffness

Figure 5–2. The primary local treatment of burns of the hand.

skin grafting at earliest possible time (when wound bed is prepared)
early movement to diminish joint stiffening

IMMEDIATE EXCISION OF FULL-THICKNESS BURNS

If the area is confined to the hand and is full-thickness destruction, anesthetic to pinprick, immediate excision is the best solution.

Figure 5–3*A* shows a full-thickness burn of the back of the hand secondary to contact with a 3000° heating element. It was excised and closed primarily on the day of injury. It healed completely by the twenty-first day, a relatively short convalescence.

The extreme temperature to which this man was exposed by history and the dry coagulated appearance of the burned skin, combined with complete lack of pain sensation to pinprick, indicated full thickness destruction. The eschar was excised to a bleeding margin of skin and deep tissue before closure.

CHEMICAL INJURY

The skin may be destroyed by strong acids or alkalis. Physical removal of the material and neutralization of the pH at the earliest possible time is the best treatment. This involves copious washing

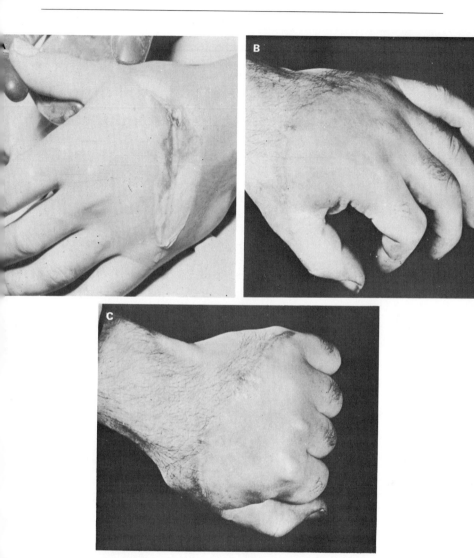

Figure 5–3. Immediate excision of a full-thickness burn. *A*, A forty-five-year-old man bumped the back of his right hand against a 3000° heating element. The skin was coagulated, white, and anesthetic. It was excised on the day of injury, and primary closure was carried out. Three weeks later, the wound was healed and his hand movements were normal. A long protracted healing period with possible joint stiffening was avoided in this case. If there is question about viability of the deep layers of skin, however, delay and local treatment with antibiotic ointment is indicated. Skin graft can be performed later, as necessary, when the depth of the destruction is recognizable. *B* and *C*, appearance two months after the treatment was instituted.

with warm water followed by appropriate neutralizing solution as soon as available. Hydrofluoric acid burns should have 10% calcium gluconate infiltrated into the area (see below).

Phosphorus burns, although infrequent in civilian practice, are common in modern warfare because of the use of this element in smoke screens, incendiary bombs, and tracer bullets. Phosphorus oxidizes in air to phosphorus pentoxide which, by taking up water, changes to phosphoric acid. The phosphorus in the wound may emit smoke when exposed to air and glow bluish green in the dark.[14]

Treat phosphorus wounds in this order:

1. Flood with warm water.
2. Physically remove phosphorus particles.
3. Alkalinize with weak sodium bicarbonate solution (two tablespoons per pint of water).

Application of 1% copper sulfate solution causes the phosphorus particles to turn black so that they are more readily recognized for removal. This solution, however, should be used with caution because copper poisoning with hemolysis of red blood cells has been reported.[14]

Figure 5–4A shows the wrist of a forty-year-old man who had been cleaning a brick wall with muriatic acid (HCl) four days earlier. The acid got beneath the cuff of his glove, burning his wrist as shown. It should have been neutralized with sodium bicarbonate, but, instead, the patient continued with his work. The areas were anesthetic to pinprick.

He was admitted to the hospital on the same day and on the following morning the areas of necrotic skin on the volar surface of the right wrist, 6 cm × 4 cm and $2\frac{1}{2}$ cm × $3\frac{1}{2}$ cm, were excised to healthy tissue and dermatome skin grafts 0.016 inch thick sutured into place and covered with a gentle pressure dressing with fluff gauze and elastic bandages.

The smaller areas of destruction on the volar surface of the left wrist were treated with bacitracin ointment and debrided surgically. Healing of the grafted areas was *per primum*, as shown in figure 5–4B, and normal wrist function followed. His period of morbidity was greatly reduced by immediate skin grafting.

Hydrofluoric acid burns are particularly dangerous owing to the destructive nature of the fluoride ion, in addition to the hydrogen-ion dehydration and corrosion which occur.

Iverson, Laub, and Madison[9] have found the local infiltration of 10% calcium gluconate to be the most effective means of neutralizing the fluoride ion. (Calcium fluoride and magnesium fluoride salts are insoluble.) From their experience with the treatment of eighty-five patients as well as animal experimentation, the following plan of

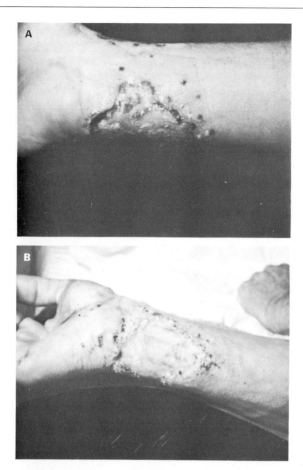

Figure 5–4. Chemical injury. *A*, appearance of the wrist of a 40-year-old man four days after being burned with muriatic acid. The patient had begun to notice a burning after about five hours of work as a result of acid getting beneath the cuff of his glove. When seen the patient's right wrist was gray and necrotic and the area was anesthetic to pinprick. *B*, appearance of the wrist twelve days after treatment with a dermatome skin graft. The graft continued to heal *per primam* without complication.

treatment for hydrofluoric acid burns is recommended:

1. Wash copiously all exposed areas with tap water. Alkaline soap can be used in conjunction with this if available.
2. Irrigate the eyes, if exposed, with a large volume of fluid.
3. Infiltrate 10% calcium gluconate subcutaneously in and around the area. The injection should be through a 30-gauge needle in small volumes which do not distend the

tissues (approximately one-half milliliter per square centimeter). The injection should be given without prior local anesthesia. Inject until the pain disappears. If the patient's pain is used as a monitor, the smallest effective amount of calcium can be given. The only exception to the use of calcium injections for hydrofluoric burns is with an exposure to less than 20% hydrogen fluoride, when no pain or skin changes are present. In these cases, an initial cleansing and close observation are recommended.

4. Iced 25% magnesium sulfate soaks should be applied to the burned areas if there is a delay in medical attention after the initial washing.
5. Following calcium gluconate injections, severe burns should be anesthetized and carefully debrided. The fingernail(s) should be removed if there is subungual exposure.
6. The patient should be carefully observed. If pain recurs, additional calcium gluconate should be administered.
7. Pulmonary edema should be anticipated if there has been inhalation of hydrogen fluoride. Parenteral steroids probably should be given, as they are with other severe pulmonary burns.

FROSTBITE

Low temperature may cause freezing of part or all of an extremity. As the body temperature drops during exposure to cold, the blood in the extremities is shunted from the arterial to the venous circulation. This is the way central body temperature is maintained. For this reason, as well as the greater heat loss peripherally, the most distal portions of the extremity are most vulnerable.

Prevention of frostbite is by far easier than treatment. Sudden blanching of the part and numbness or pain which subsides are the danger signs which should be quickly heeded. Warming of the hand in the armpit or other warm area of the body is very useful to reverse incipient changes, but rapid thawing in hot water (40° to 42° C) three to five degrees above body temperature to restore circulation quickly in established cases is indicated.

Frostbite has been classified into four degrees similar to burns:[16]

1. First degree (erythema)
2. Second degree (blistering)
3. Third degree (partial gangrene)
4. Fourth degree (complete loss of the part)

Washburn,[18] whose excellent treatise should be read by all interested, points out the difficulty in immediate assessment and advocates de-

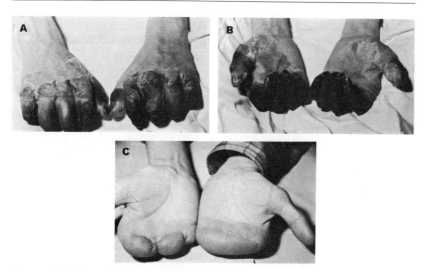

Figure 5–5. Frostbite. *A* and *B*, the hands of a fifty-four-year-old man one week after he had lain in snow at —10°F for about three hours. Rapid thawing was not employed and the fingers were all necrotic, requiring amputation. The thumbs were saved. *C*, the appearance three months later following amputation of the fingers.

termining superficial or deep injury only. Skin and subcutaneous tissue involvement is considered superficial frostbite; the deep structures are still pliable in this degree of injury. Complete solid freezing is classified as deep injury.

Because of the experimental work of Fuhrman and Crismon,[6] Finneran and Shumacker,[5] and Entin and Baxter,[4] it is now agreed that thawing should be carried out rapidly by immersion in a hot water bath of 40° to 42° C (104° to 108° F) until the part becomes pink.[10, 18] This usually occurs within twenty minutes. The thawing phase is painful and requires medication. According to Mills,[10] rubbing a frostbitten portion of the body with snow is as illogical as putting a burned portion of the body in the oven! The value of anticoagulation and sympathetic blocks is less well established, but it probably has value in maintaining circulation in small vessels damaged by freezing. Shumacker,[16] DeJong,[3] and Weatherley-White[19] have shown that dextran is beneficial in diminishing the extent of cold injury in animals.

The hands of a fifty-four-year-old man are shown in figure 5–5*A* one week after freezing in snow at —10° F. Rapid thawing was not employed. His fingers were completely necrotic, requiring amputation. The thumbs survived, as is often the case. After finger amputation the wounds were closed by abdominal pedicle flaps, as

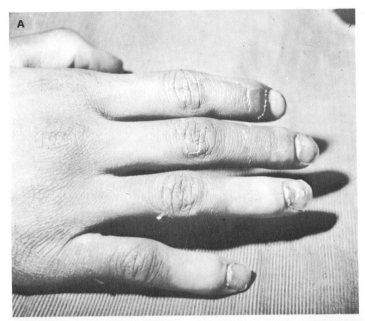

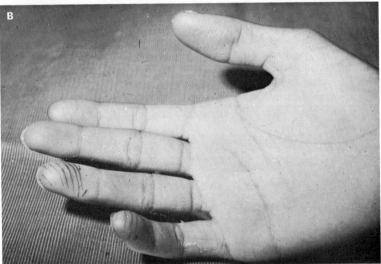

Figure 5–6. Frostbite. *A*, a fourteen-year-old young man played football with his hands bare for forty-five minutes in a temperature of —4°F and his fingers were numb and white upon presentation. Treatment in the emergency room by an astute resident consisted of bathing the patient's hands in hot water at 42°C (180°F) for fifteen minutes followed by dextran and repeated sympathetic nerve blocks. He was hospitalized for ten days. Severe blistering occurred, most marked on the ring and small fingers, which was followed by crust formation. *B*, the left hand four weeks after injury. Sensation was limited over the tips of the ring and small fingers, but this later cleared. The ring and small fingers probably were saved by the rigorous treatment.

shown in figure 5–5*B*. Some finger function might have been preserved by rapid thawing.

Figure 5–6 shows the result of rigorous treatment of less severe frostbite in a young man fourteen years of age.

Bibliography

1. Artz, Curtis P., and Moncrief, John A.: *The Treatment of Burns*, 2d ed., p. 228 (Philadelphia: W. B. Saunders Co., 1969).

2. Baxter, Charles: Homografts and heterografts as a biologic dressing in the treatment of thermal injury. Paper presented at First Annual Congress of Society of German Plastic Surgeons, 28 September 1970, Munich.

3. DeJong, Pieter; Golding, Michael R.; Sawyer, Philip N.; and Wesolowski, Sigmund A.: The role of regional sympathectomy in the early management of cold injury, Surg. Gynecol. Obstet. 115:45–48, 1962.

4. Entin, Martin A., and Baxter, Hamilton: Influence of rapid warming on frostbite in experimental animals, Plast. Reconstr. Surg. 9:511–24, 1952.

5. Finneran, Joseph C., and Shumacker, Harris B., Jr.: Studies in experimental frostbite: V. Further evaluation of early treatment, Surg. Gynecol. Obstet. 90:430–38, 1950.

6. Fuhrman, Frederick A., and Crismon, J. M.: Studies on gangrene following cold injury: II. General course of events in rabbit feet and ears following untreated cold injury, J. Clin. Invest. 26:236, 1947.

7. Hermann, Gilbert; Schechter, David C.; Owens, J. Cuthbert; and Starzl, Thomas E.: The problem of frostbite in civilian medical practice, Surg. Clin. North Am. 43, no. 2:519–36, April 1963.

8. Hurley, J. V.; Ham, Kathryn N.; and Ryan, G. B.: The mechanism of the delayed prolonged phase of increased vascular permeability in mild thermal injury in the rat, J. Pathol. 94:1–12, 1967.

9. Iverson, Ronald E.; Laub, Donald R.; and Madison, Mitchell S.: Hydrofluoric acid burns, Plast. Reconstr. Surg. 48:107–12, 1971.

10. Mills, William J., Jr.: Frostbite: A method of management including rapid thawing, Northwest Med. 65:119–25, 1966.

11. Moncrief, John A.; Switzer, Walter E.; and Rose, Lawrence, R.: Primary excision and grafting in the treatment of third-degree burns of the dorsum of the hand, Plast. Reconstr. Surg. 33:305–16, 1964.

12. O'Neill, James A., Jr.; Grosfeld, Jay L.: and Boles, E. Thomas, Jr.: The extended use of skin homografts, Arch. Surg. 99:263–68, 1969.

13. Procaine Skin Dressings (Burn Treatment Skin Bank, Inc., 2430 East Washington Street, Phoenix, Arizona 85034).
14. Rabinowitch, I. M.: Treatment of phosphorous burns (with a note on acute phosphorous poisoning), Can. Med. Assoc. J. 48:291–96, 1943.
15. Shuck, Jerry M.; Moncrief, John A.; and Monafo, William W.: The management of burns, Curr. Probl. Surg., February 1969.
16. Shumacker, Harris B., Jr.: Sympathectomy in the treatment of frostbite, Surg. Gynecol. Obstet. 93:727–34, 1951.
17. Summerlin, William T.; Walder, Arnold I.; and Moncrief, John A.: White phosphorus burns and massive hemolysis, J. Trauma 7:476–84, 1967.
18. Washburn, Bradford: Frostbite: What it is—how to prevent it—emergency treatment, New Engl. J. Med. 266:974–89, 1962.
19. Weatherley-White, R. C. A.; Paton, Bruce, C.; and Sjostrom, Bjorn: Experimental studies in cold injury: III. Observations on the treatment of frostbite, Plast. Reconstr. Surg. 36:10–18, 1965.

CHAPTER 6

Electrical Injury

ABSTRACT

The passage of high voltage electrical currents through the tissues of the body can cause death by producing ventricular fibrillation or respiratory paralysis. It also can cause deep and widespread local tissue destruction by its direct effect and by the high temperatures produced. These temperatures may be up to several thousand degrees centigrade when the current arcs. Seventy-five percent of patients with electrical injury have burns of one or both hands.

First aid consists of freeing the patient from the current at the earlier possible time. Ideally, the current should be shut off. The danger of arcing should be kept in mind when working near high tension lines. The distance a current will arc is several centimeters for each ten thousand volts, and it will extend for many feet once the arc is established.

Local destruction (coagulation necrosis) is deep and extensive, involving whole portions of the extremity, making the danger of renal failure from hemoglobinemia greater than with surface burns. Urine output should be kept at 50 ml per hour to prevent this. The wounds should be debrided early and repeatedly until a healthy base is obtained; then coverage by free graft or pedicle graft is indicated.

Pitfalls

1. *Renal shutdown, caused by greater deep tissue destruction than recognized on surface*
2. *Vascular impairment because of swelling and constriction, which requires early fasciotomy and debridement*
3. *Loss of deep tissues by unnecessary delay of debridement and grafting*

The effects of high voltage electrical currents passing through the human body are multiple and severe. Death may be caused by ventricular fibrillation or respiratory paralysis. Fractures and dislocations may occur as muscle groups are thrown into tetanic contraction. The destruction of local tissue may be widespread and deep. The passage of current through the tissue as well as the intense heat generated may cause coagulation necrosis and secondary thrombosis of the blood vessels. Clothing may ignite, and the patient may fall, causing further injury.

The resistance of various tissues to the flow of current, in ascending order, is nerve, blood, muscle, skin, tendon fat, and finally bone.[1,2] The only poor conductor in the body is bone. Much additional damage occurs from the secondary thrombosis of vessels damaged by the current. This damage may also cause rupture, producing secondary hemorrhage. Electrical injuries cause 1,100 deaths in the United States annually,[6] and have accounted for 3 percent of the cases admitted to one major burn center according to Baxter,[2] and for 7 percent according to Skoog.[9]

The degree of destruction is related to the amount and duration of the current and the resistance and size of the tissue mass through which it passes. Fingers may be burned away and a forearm badly damaged while the greater mass of the trunk shows no untoward effect if ventricular fibrillation or respiratory paralysis has not occurred. If the current exits through the feet, toes and foot may be damaged, usually less than the point of entry.

For prophylaxis, it should be remembered that high tension lines will arc several centimeters for each ten thousand volts[9] and that once the arc is established it will persist for many feet. The arcing temperature may be as high as 4000°C.

Seventy-five percent of patients with electrical injury have burns of one or both hands. Contact itself causes tight closure of grasp and flexion of the wrist, inducing further arcing and destruction of volar tissues of hand and forearm.[9]

Electrical destruction of tissue, in contrast to external heat injury, does not diminish rapidly as the tissues are penetrated. Instead, the injury penetrates deep beneath the surface in the path of flow of the current. Whole portions of arm, forearm, and hand may be completely necrosed by the effects of the current. Electrical forces have been called manifestations of the ultimate structure of matter.[3]

The surgical care of the patient who has received electrical injuries is very taxing because of the extent of the injury, the difficulty of determining the limits of the injury, and the changes that may be progressive, especially those from secondary vascular thrombosis. Vascular damage consists of injury to intima and media. Media necrosis may lead to secondary hemorrhage (Robinson, Masters, and Forrest[8]).

An outline of treatment is as follows:

    1. First aid in this order:

        Current shut off. (If attempts to remove the victim from the current with a nonconductor are made, beware of arcing.)

Mouth-to-mouth respiration, cardiac massage, and defibrillation by shock if necessary and available

2. Systemic:

Fluid and electrolyte replacement to keep urinary output high (more than 50 ml per hour) and prevent globin cast production in renal tubules secondary to muscle injury and hemolysis[4]

Broad spectrum antibiotic

Dextran

Heparin

Tetanus prophylaxis

Electrocardiogram and electroencephalogram

3. Local:

Cleansing and local application of Sulfamylon or antibiotic ointment

Early debridement and fasciotomy (repeat as necessary)

Skin grafting (free or pedicle) as soon as blood supply of bed of recipient area will support it

Freeing the victim from the current promptly, mouth-to-mouth respiration, cardiac massage, and defibrillation may be lifesaving if used in time. Systemic treatment once the patient has survived should emphasize fluid and electrolyte replacement to keep the urine output high and protect the kidneys from myoglobin cast production. Antibiotics and specific tetanus prophylaxis are important. Dextran and possibly heparin should be given to prevent further thrombosis of vessels. Figure 6–1 shows a thirteen-year-old boy with extensive electrical injury to his right hand and forearm whose radial and ulnar arteries thrombosed on the fifth post-injury day. Whether heparin might have prevented thrombosis is open to question. It was not used because active debridement was being carried out and the danger of hemorrhage was present.

Local treatment should emphasize sterility, prevention of infection, debridement, and skin grafting. Peterson favors early excision.[7] In my experience, debridement often needs to be repeated because of difficulty in accurately recognizing the demarcation between injured and healthy tissue and the progression of vascular thrombosis. Skoog[9] has had similar experience.

Mafenide acetate (Sulfamylon cream), gentamicin sulfate (Garamycin), or another suitable antibiotic ointment serves very well for local treatment.

Skin grafting and pedicle flap coverage should be done at the earliest possible time to preserve essential deep structures, although there is difficulty recognizing and separating devitalized from healthy tissue.

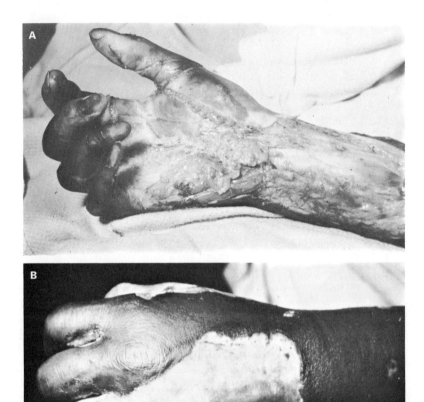

Figure 6-1. Electrical injury. *A* and *B* show the original appearance of the right hand and forearm of a thirteen-year-old boy who attempted to pull a telephone from a high tension wire. Note the extreme destruction of the volar surfaces of the hand and forearm. There were less severe burns of both feet (points of exit of current). The wounds were debrided and left open six times before closure with an abdominal pedicle flap to cover denuded tendons. During the successive debridements, the radial and ulnar arteries were preserved five days, but then lost to thrombosis. Dextran but not heparin was used during the debridement stage. Two years later, the patient had pinch between thumb and index finger, but was very self-conscious of his deformed hand.

In practice, as debridement is carried out in severe cases, it has seemed that the deep structures tend to lose viability on exposure so that further debridement is needed at the next stage. The problem is to cover vital structures with pedicle tissue at the earliest possible time that this can be done and still not have severe breakdown of tissue beneath the flap. This is a decision which taxes the most experienced. There are no easy solutions or strict guidelines in the severe cases.

After adequate skin and subcutaneous tissue coverage has been accomplished, reconstructive procedures to enhance prehension and sensation may be possible. Each case must be individualized because there is no standard pattern of destruction.

Late sequelae may occur, according to Baxter.[2] These may be disturbances of neurological function, cataracts, or gastrointestinal complaints.

Bibliography

1. Artz, Curtis P., and Moncrief, John A.: *The Treatment of Burns*, 2d ed., pp. 214–16 (Philadelphia: W. B. Saunders Co., 1969).
2. Baxter, Charles R.: Present concepts in the management of major electrical injury, Surg. Clin. North Am. 50, no. 6: 1401–18, December 1970.
3. Dale, R. H.: Electrical accidents: A discussion with illustrative cases, Br. J. Plast. Surg. 7: 44–66, 1954.
4. DiVincenti, Frank C.; Moncrief, John A.; and Pruitt, Basil A, Jr.: Electrical injuries: A review of 65 cases, J. Trauma 9: 497–507, 1969.
5. Kouwenhoven, W. B.: Effects of electricity on the human body, Electrical Engineering 68: 199–203, 1949.
6. Mills, William, Jr.; Switzer, Walter E.; and Moncrief, John A.: Electrical injuries, J.A.M.A. 195: 852–54, 1966.
7. Peterson, Rex A.: Electrical burns of the hand: Treatment by early excision, J. Bone Joint Surg. 48-A: 407–24, 1966.
8. Robinson, David W.; Masters, Frank W.; and Forrest, William J.: Electrical burns: A review and analysis of 33 cases, Surgery 57: 385–90, 1965.
9. Skoog, Tord: Electrical injuries, J. Trauma 10: 816–30, 1970.

CHAPTER 7

Fingertip Injury, Amputation, and Replantation of Severed Parts of an Extremity

ABSTRACT

Fingertip injuries are treated best by local flaps if at all possible. The severity of the problem of closure depends upon the relative length of the bone and soft tissues and the amount of pulp tissue which is lost. I favor retaining bone length. Free skin grafts are satisfactory if a soft tissue bed remains. Skin from the ulnar border of the hand (hypothenar eminence) may be utilized. This should be placed away from the pulp of the fingertip if possible. Local advancement flaps, such as V-Y or volar advancement, are useful when the bone and soft tissues are of equal length. When the bone projects, thenar or cross-finger pedicles are usually necessary. Remote pedicle coverage, such as from the abdomen or deltopectoral area, may be necessary in extreme cases. If sensation in the pedicle tissue is not adequate, island pedicle tissue from a normal finger can be added later to overcome this. The simplest procedure which maintains length and gives good soft tissue at the tip should be chosen in each individual case.

Amputations of more than the tips of the fingers should be treated according to the same general principles as fingertip injuries. Volar tissue makes the best closure when available. Flexor profundus tendons should be allowed to retract. They should not be reattached to the middle or proximal phalanges.

Entire ray amputation (phalanges and metacarpal) for injuries is justifiable, especially if the patient does not use heavy tools in his work. An adjacent marginal digit can be moved to the position of the amputated ray in the case of ring or long finger loss. This gives good appearance and function.

Replantation of an upper extremity by vascular, tendon, and nerve repair is practical in selected cases. Primary treatment is outlined as well as the factors which might make it successful if carried out within six hours after injury.

Pitfalls

1. *Tender amputation stump caused by neuroma formation*
2. *Tender amputation stump caused by lack of soft sub-cutaneous tissue*
3. *Amputated digit too short for function. (This is not frequent if sensation is satisfactory.)*

Recommended for Early Transfer to a Medical Center

Complete, sharp severance of the major portion of an extremity in an otherwise healthy patient seen early after injury if not in shock and having no other serious injury. (The extremity should be packed in ice and saline and sent with the patient.)

The normal fingertip is soft and pliable, and its tactile sense exquisite. These qualities should be retained and restored as much as possible. Failure involves lack of adequate soft tissue or inadequate sensation. Usually the relative length of the remaining bone and soft tissues and the obliquity of the destruction (amount of pulp missing) determine what can be done. The digits used most in apposition with the thumb—normally the more radially located digits—are of greatest importance to hand function.

The use of local skin for closure is best, when this can be accomplished. The nerve endings of the local tissues are most suited for the required sensation, and the presence of dermal ridges in the skin texture here is best. Metcalf and Whalen[15] and others have emphasized this. Viable local flaps should be preserved with this in mind whenever possible and bone length preserved to maintain as much of the length of the digit as possible. If remaining adjacent tissue can be brought to the apposable portion of the digit, this is highly desirable. Free skin grafts provide adequate closure when adequate subcutaneous padding remains, in spite of their limited sensory return. Placement of the free graft in a less utilized tactile area is desirable. Littler,[13] Flint and Harrison,[5] and Beasley[2] advocate this and offer special methods of carrying it out. Lie, Magargle, and Posch[12] utilize a free graft of full thickness skin from the hypothenar area, a method I also find useful. The tight arrangement of the tissues of the finger end, with rather rigid fibrous attachments between volar skin and deep structures, complicates the problem.

The following outline of procedures is offered on the basis of relative bone and soft tissue length and the amount of pulp tissue remaining.

1. Soft tissue longer than bone (viable local skin flaps)
   a. Primary closure
   b. Free skin graft:

deep partial or full-thickness free skin graft, placed
in less utilized tactile area if possible

2. Soft tissues and bone same length (guillotine amputation)
   a. Bilateral V-Y advancement (Kutler[11]) or single V-Y
      (Atasoy et al.[1])
   b. Volar flap advancement (Littler,[13] O'Brien,[17] Snow,[18]
      Beasley[2])
   c. Pedicle:
      cross-finger
      thenar
      remote

3. Bone longer than soft tissues or extensive pulp injury
   (oblique pulp removal)
   a. Pedicle (see chapter 4):
      cross-finger
      thenar
      dorsal flap (Flint and Harrison[5])
      island
      remote (abdomen, chest, arm)

When the soft tissues exceed the bone in length there are fewer
problems. Direct soft tissue closure may be possible. A small free
skin graft (deep partial or full thickness) usually works well, although
the size and shape of the defect and exposure of deep structures
influence the type of repair which should be done. Hypothenar skin
may be used.[12]

V-Y ADVANCEMENT

When local skin flaps do not exist and the bone and soft tissues
are divided in the same plane, the method of Kutler[11] has much
to commend it. Local tissue is still utilized (figure 7−1). The V-Y
advancement from either side prevents the formation of "dog-ears"
by moving the excess lateral tissue further distally into a useful
position to cover the tip. In this way, the bone end is covered with
soft tissue and skin with suitable nerve endings. Some of the normal
tapered contour of the fingertip is thus restored. I have had good
results with this technique, although sensory acuity has been reduced.
The triangular flaps should not be undercut; care must be taken to
preserve blood supply and sensation as much as possible. The flaps
should be brought together as far volarward as possible. Under some
circumstances, if necessary, they may be supplemented with a small
free graft placed according to the principles of fingertip treatment,
that is, away from apposable tactile areas. Fisher[4] advocates rounding

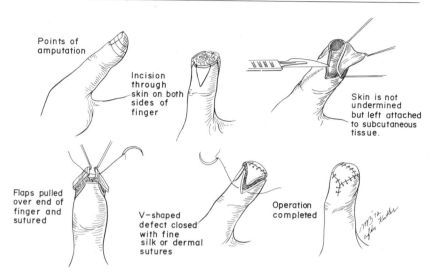

Points of amputation

Incision through skin on both sides of finger

Skin is not undermined but left attached to subcutaneous tissue.

Flaps pulled over end of finger and sutured

V-shaped defect closed with fine silk or dermal sutures

Operation completed

Figure 7–1. Kutler method of fingertip closure when bone and soft tissues are the same length. The excess tissues at either side ("dog-ears") are advanced to cover the tip (V-Y advancement). The diamond-shaped flaps are not undercut, and thus their nerve and blood supply are partially maintained. This technique has been modified by Atasoy et al.[1] to a single volar flap. The principle has been adapted to other areas of the body (see Trevaskis et al., chapter 4, page 74). (Redrawn, with permission, from Kutler, A new method for finger tip amputation, J.A.M.A., 133 : 29–30, 1947. Copyright 1947, American Medical Association.)

of the lateral bone edges with a rongeur to minimize angulation and tension of the subcutaneous tissues. Figure 7–2 shows a good result five months after closure with the Kutler technique, although sensation is still reduced. Atasoy et al.[1] have modified this technique to a single volar flap.

VOLAR FLAP ADVANCEMENT

Advancement of a portion of the volar tissues of the finger for fingertip closure has been advocated by Littler,[13] O'Brien,[16] and Beasley.[2]

Advancement of the entire volar portion of the digit has been advocated by Snow[18] for amputations through a portion of the distal phalanx (figure 7–3). By flexing the finger, the freed volar flap of the finger is brought over the end of the digit, sutured in that position, and held in flexion by plaster for three weeks. The

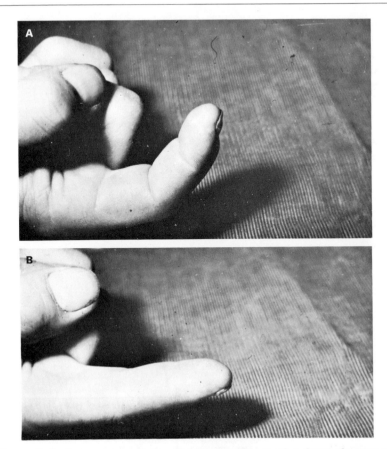

Figure 7–2. Appearance of the right index finger of a forty-six-year-old man five months after it was amputated transversely at the middle of the fingernail by a punch press. Closure was carried out by the Kutler method immediately after the injury. This is an unusually good result and the restored convexity of the fingertip is noteworthy as is his 3 mm 2-point discrimination.

finger is then freed and the patient allowed to stretch his finger straight. These techniques of advancement can bring intact sensory skin to the tip of the digit where it is most needed. The volar tissues of the adult finger can be advanced approximately one centimeter if they are freed from the attachment to the flexor tendon tunnel. Snow has advocated bilateral, midlateral incision to accomplish this. I utilize a unilateral incision to maintain blood supply to the dorsal area. The volar attachments to the tendon tunnel and Cleland's ligament can be freed bilaterally through a single midlateral incision;

this leaves the dorsal branches on the opposite side to supply the dorsum of the finger.

Figure 7–3 shows the use of volar advancement to close the tip of a finger with a sensitive scar. After removal of the sensitive area at the tip of the amputation stump at the middle of the middle phalanx, the volar tissues were elevated through a single midlateral incision and advanced one centimeter for closure. The tissues came together well, as shown in figure 7–3C, D, and E. The finger extended satisfactorily in a few weeks.

PALMAR PEDICLE FLAP (THENAR)

The utilization of palmar or thenar tissue (see chapter 4, page 78) to repair a volar defect on the distal portion of the finger, reported by Gatewood[7] in 1926, has been widely utilized. This very useful method (figure 7–4) may be followed by troublesome inter-phalangeal joint stiffness in some people because of the rather complete immobilization in flexion, especially in older people. This can be avoided by periarticular infiltration of corticosteroids, such as triamcinolone acetonide, prophylactically (see chapter 3). The thenar pedicle restores soft tissue padding well. With time, fairly good sensory return occurs, even though the nerve supply is completely detached during the process of transfer.

The finger needs to be bandaged in flexion for about three weeks to avoid tension on the flap. The donor site is covered with a free graft from the forearm at the time of construction of the pedicle.

CROSS-FINGER PEDICLE FLAP

Utilization of the tissues of an adjacent finger by means of a pedicle flap (chapter 4, page 79) has become popular since the reports of Gurdin and Pangman[8] and Tempest.[20] There is less difficulty with joint stiffness than with the palmar or thenar flap since immobilization of one finger to another is less rigid than immobilization to the palm or thenar area. Soft tissue padding is supplied over bone or tendon, and nerve regeneration is usually quite good. Possible injury to the normal donor finger is a small hazard. These flaps should be made larger than the defect they are to cover to allow for shrinkage, and care should be taken to avoid kinking.

The fingers are bandaged together for three weeks. The donor area is covered with a free skin graft at the time of construction, usually from the forearm.

Figure 7–4 shows a case in which two fingers were amputated. This was treated by a thenar pedicle to one and a cross-finger pedicle to the other.

NEUROVASCULAR ISLAND PEDICLE

The transfer of a block of tissue with an intact nerve and blood supply, but no intervening bridge of skin (see chapter 4, page 80), is a clever idea which has specific application in hand surgery. Before the development of this technique it was considered that the

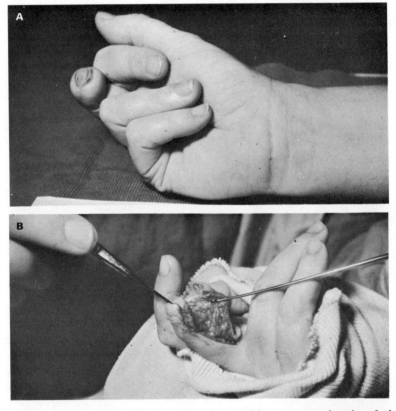

Figure 7–3. Volar flap advancement. *A,* sensitive scar at the tip of the amputated right long finger of a thirty-five-year-old woman who lost the portion through the middle phalanx nine months earlier. *B,* elevation of the volar flap through a single midlateral incision. *C, D,* and *E,* after excision of the cicatrix and elevation of the volar tissues, they are advanced as shown.

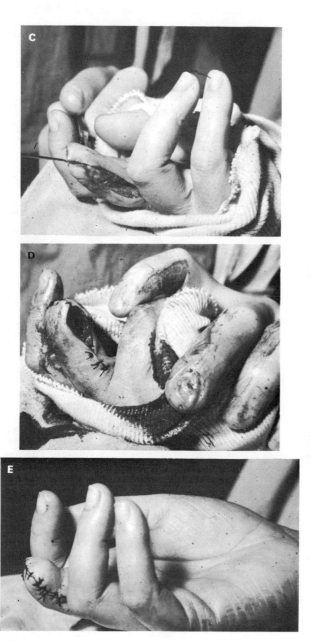

Figure 7–3 (con't.)

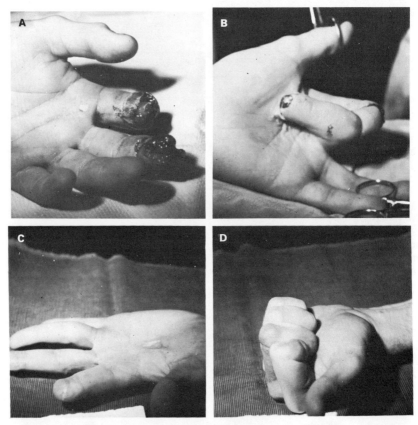

Figure 7–4. Palmar pedicle flap and cross-finger pedicle flap. *A*, a nineteen-year-old patient caught his left index and long fingers between a tractor and farm machine, sustaining the amputations shown. *B*, the long fingertip was covered by a thenar pedicle and the index finger by a cross-finger flap from the dorsum of the long finger, "piggyback fashion." One-half milliliter triamcinolone (5 mgm) was injected into periarticular tissues of the middle joints of each of the immobilized fingers. The fingers were detached at four weeks. *C* and *D* show the result two months later.

venous return in the neurovascular bundle of the finger wound not be adequate. Subsequent experience, however, has proved that it is adequate if the vessels and nerves are very gently dissected free during the transfer. Completely normal sensation can be restored to an anesthetic area by this means, since no interruption of the main nerve to the area is necessary during the transfer. (Sensation in the pedicle is not interrupted.) In addition, the vascularity of the recipient area is increased. In my experience this technique is useful to restore sensation and also to increase the circulation of a digit.

When sensation is shifted from one area of the hand to another, the patient must relearn the new location. This poses a problem for some people, but most are able to do it effectively.

The development of the technique for transfer of the neurovascular island pedicle to restore sensation was made by Littler[13] in America and Moberg[16] in Sweden. Both of these men were greatly influenced by the previous work of Sterling Bunnell,[3] who had transferred an index finger on its neurovascular pedicles without intervening skin, at Letterman Hospital in 1951. Dr. Bunnell gave credit for the previous use of vascular pedicles to Gersuny, in 1887, and Esser, in 1917. Hilgenfeldt[9] had described transfer of the long finger to thumb position, utilizing an intervening skin bridge in addition to the vessels.

Frackelton and Teasley,[6] Tubiana,[21] and others made early contributions to the technique of island pedicle transfer, demonstrating the practicality of the procedure.

The technique can be utilized to bring normal sensation to the dominant portion of the hand. It can also be utilized to cover large pulp losses on the index finger or thumb, either primarily or secondarily (Frackelton and Teasley,[6] Sullivan et al.[19]).

Extensive loss of pulp tissue may best be treated by an island pedicle flap. For less extensive losses, volar flap advancement is a more direct approach. Any technique which utilizes local tissue and does not involve alteration of another portion of the hand is especially desirable.

REMOTE PEDICLES

The use of tissue from a remote area, such as the abdominal or chest wall (deltopectoral) area, may be necessary in extreme cases. Sensation of the skin supplied by this type of pedicle is limited. This, however, can be overcome by the use of an island pedicle to supply sensation at a later operation if necessary.

TREATMENT OF DIVIDED NERVES

The problem of treating divided nerves is not completely solved. At the tip of the finger the nerves are too small to deal with individually and the retention or restoration of soft tissue to provide padding is the best assurance against neuroma formation. When the digital nerves are recognizable, as at the base of the distal phalanx or further proximal, they should be ligated with nonabsorbable ligature, injected with corticosteroid, and buried as deeply as possible in soft tissue.

FINGERNAIL

The normal fingernail bed should be preserved when possible. Lacerations should be sutured with fine absorbable suture material, such as 5–0 chromic catgut. Small fragments may lead to deformity and are best excised. Head loupe magnification is very helpful.

AMPUTATIONS

The same general principles apply to amputations of fingers that apply to fingertip injuries. As much bone length should be retained as possible after rounding off ragged bone edges. Here, too, local flaps make the best closure if enough soft tissue remains to accomplish this. Volar tissue, when sufficient, serves best over the amputated ends. Dorsal tissue is second choice, and pedicle tissue third choice. Nerve ends should be ligated with nonabsorbable ligatures and allowed to retract beneath other soft tissues for protection, as mentioned previously. Divided profundus tendons should be allowed to retract into the palm. They should not be sutured to the volar surface of the middle or the proximal phalanx because this frequently interferes with the excursion of the profundus tendons of the other fingers. The latter is due to the presence, in most people, of one common muscle belly for all four profundus tendons.

Working men need the full width of their palms in handling large tools. For this reason, a metacarpal head may have value to a workman, even though the digit is amputated at the M-P joint. In women, however, and in men who do not use their hands for heavy work, the metacarpal head or the entire metacarpal may be removed to improve appearance. When this is done for the long or ring finger, the adjacent marginal digit along with the metacarpal can be transposed to the base of the amputated metacarpal by the experienced operator. This improves appearance, closes the gap between fingers, and prevents overlapping of the remaining fingers by aligning and fixing all remaining metacarpals adjacent to one another. When the operation is well carried out, the resulting three-fingered hand has a near-normal appearance (see figure 11–16, page 235).

REPLANTATION OF SEVERED PARTS OF AN EXTREMITY

The reattachment of a portion of an extremity, with the exception of skin only and, rarely, a portion of a distal phalanx, requires that the continuity of the arteries and veins be restored. Buncke and Schulz,[22] working with monkeys, in some instances found that portions of the distal phalanx have survived if the skin and subcutaneous tissue is reattached accurately but without vascular anastomosis. In my own practice, this is an infrequent occurrence in view of the number of times I have had to remove black portions of digits which had been reattached by others. However, the skin from any recently severed part, if not severely traumatized, can be used successfully as a free skin graft.

In addition to survival following vascular reconstruction, usefulness of a reattached part depends upon restored nerve, tendon, and joint function. Without these, restoration is not worthwhile in the upper extremity. Replantation of the major portion of an arm has been shown to be practical since first carried out successfully by Malt and McKhann[27] in 1962. In a review by Engber and Hardin[24] twenty-five of thirty-five reported cases (71 percent) had useful function. Eight of the ten cases with less than a good result had been reamputated. Some poor results probably have not been reported. The good result reported by Rosenkrantz et al.,[30] involving the left arm of a two-year-old child severed through the proximal humerus, demonstrates the great regenerative ability of nerves in the young age group. This child regained remarkably good function of the replanted left arm and hand. Long term follow up on two adult patients lead Harris and Malt[25] to conclude that human upper limb replantation is justified in selected cases.

Vascular anastomosis is more readily carried out in the proximal portion of the upper extremity where the vessels are larger. Nerve regeneration following repair at this level, however, is less good. Distally, the blood vessels become smaller and vascular restoration is more difficult, but the results of nerve repair are better. The most distal level at which microscopic vascular repair is practical at the present time is probably at the level of the palm, although isolated cases of replacement of individual digits are recorded. Two recent reports[23, 29] give more than a fifty percent survival rate for replanted digits, many of which regained useful function.

Replantation of an extremity or any significant part of it requiring vascular, nerve, and tendon repair is a major undertaking which should be attempted only in a center with many special services and skilled personnel available. It requires team effort with one group treating the patient at the same time the other group works with the detached extremity, which must be cooled, cleansed, debrided, and its vessels prepared for anastomosis. An artery of the detached part should be perfused with cooled, lactated Ringer's solution containing heparin and a nonirritating antibiotic, such as penicillin, to which the patient is not allergic.

Success will depend upon:

1. No serious associated injury to the patient or the opposite extremity
2. Sharp severance of the extremity
3. Minimal contamination
4. Good preservation of the detached member
5. Short time-lapse between injury and reestablishment of circulation (less than six hours)
6. Cooling of the detached member (iced saline 0° to −4°C)
7. Age and good health of the patient
8. Psychological reaction of the patient and family

The clinical aspects of restoring limbs are given by Malt[26] and Malt, Remensnyder, and Harris.[28] First aid treatment of a patient with a detached extremity is:

1. Control hemorrhage, check respiration, and treat for shock.
2. Recover detached extremity and cool with ice.
3. Contact and alert medical center to problem.
4. Arrange transportation.

The final decision regarding an attempt at replantation, with all variables being considered, must be made when the patient arrives at the medical center.

Bibliography

1. Atasoy, Erdogan; Ioakimidis, Evangelos; Kasdan, Morton L.; Kutz, Joseph E.; and Kleinert, Harold E.: Reconstruction of the amputated finger tip with a triangular volar flap: A new surgical procedure, J. Bone Joint Surg. 52-A:921–26, 1970.
2. Beasley, Robert W.: Principles and techniques of resurfacing operations for hand surgery, Surg. Clin. North Am. 47, no. 2: 389–413, April 1967.
3. Bunnell, Sterling, Digit transfer by neurovascular pedicle, J. Bone Joint Surg. 34-A:772–74, 1952.
4. Fisher, Richard H.: The Kutler method of repair of finger-tip amputations, J. Bone Joint Surg. 49-A:317–21, 1967.
5. Flint, Michael H., and Harrison, Stewart H.: A local neurovascular flap to repair loss of digital pulp, Br. J. Plast. Surg. 18:156–63, 1965.
6. Frackelton, William H., and Teasley, Jack L.: Neurovascular island pedicle—extension in usage, J. Bone Joint Surg. 44-A: 1069–72, 1962.
7. Gatewood, M. D.: A plastic repair of finger defects without hospitalization, J.A.M.A. 87:1479, 1926.
8. Gurdin, Michael, and Pangman, W. John: The repair of surface

defects of fingers by transdigital flaps, Plast. Reconstr. Surg. 5:368–71, 1950.

9. Hilgenfeldt, Otto: *Operativer Daumenersatz*, pp. 32–37 (Stuttgart: Ferdinand Enke Verlag, 1950).
10. Hueston, John: Local flap repair of fingertip injuries, Plast. Reconstr. Surg. 37:349–50, 1966.
11. Kutler, William: A new method for finger tip amputation, J.A.M.A. 133:29–30, 1947.
12. Lie, Kim K.: Magargle, Ronald K.: and Posch, Joseph L.: Free full-thickness skin grafts from the palm to cover defects of the fingers, J. Bone Joint Surg. 52-A:599–61, 1970.
13. Littler, J. William (ed.): Principles of reconstructive surgery of the hand, in The Hand and Upper Extremity, p. 1638, pt. 3 of Converse, John Marquis (ed.): *Reconstructive Plastic Surgery: Principles and Procedures in Correction, Reconstruction and Transplantation*, vol. 4 (Philadelphia: W. B. Saunders Co., 1964).
14. Littler, J. William: Neurovascular skin island transfer in reconstructive hand surgery, Trans. Int. Soc. Plast. Surg. 2:175–78, 1960.
15. Metcalf, William, and Whalen, William P.: Salvage of the injured distal phalanx: Plan of care and analysis of 369 cases, Clin. Orthop. 13:114–23, 1959.
16. Moberg, Eric: Discussion of Donal Brooks: The place of nerve-grafting in orthopaedic surgery, J. Bone Joint Surg. 37-A:305, 326, 1955.
17. O'Brien, Bernard: Neurovascular pedicle transfers in the hand, Aust. N.Z. J. Surg. 35:1–11, 1965.
18. Snow, John Wesley: The use of a volar flap for repair of fingertip amputations: A preliminary report, Plast. Reconstr. Surg. 40:163–68, 1967.
19. Sullivan, J. G.; Kelleher, J. C.; Baibak, G. J.; Dean, R. K.; and Pinkner, L. D.: The primary application of an island pedicle flap in thumb and index finger injuries, Plast. Reconstr. Surg. 39:488–92, 1967.
20. Tempest, Michael N.: Cross-finger flaps in the treatment of injuries of the finger tip, Plast. Reconstr. Surg. 9:205–22, 1952.
21. Tubiana, R., and Duparc, J.: Restoration of sensibility in the hand by neurovascular skin island transfer, J. Bone Joint Surg. 43-B:474–80, 1961.

REPLANTATION

22. Buncke, Harry J., and Schulz, Werner P.: Experimental digital amputation and reimplantation, Plast. Reconstr. Surg. 36:62–70, 1965.
23. Chen Chung-Wei, Dr.: Replantation of severed fingers.

The Research Laboratory for the Replantation of Severed Limbs, the No. 6 Peoples Hospital of Shanghai, Shanghai, the Peoples Republic of China.
Address given at the annual meeting of The American Society For Surgery of The Hand, Dallas, Texas, Jan. 16, 1974.

24. Engber, William D., and Hardin, Creighton A.: Replantation of extremities, Surg. Gynecol. Obstet. 132:901–16, 1971.

25. Harris, William H. and Malt, Ronald A.: Late results of human limb replantation, J. of Trauma 14:44–52, 1974.

26. Malt, Ronald A.: Clinical aspects of restoring limbs, Advances Surg. 2:19–33, 1966.

27. Malt, Ronald A., and McKhann, Charles F.: Replantation of severed arms, J.A.M.A. 189:716–22, 1964.

28. Malt, Ronald A.; Remensnyder, John P.; and Harris, William H.: Long-term utility of replanted arms, Ann. Surg. 176:334–42, 1972.

29. O'Brien, B.M. and MacLeod, A.M.: Replantation surgery in the upper limb. Proc. Roy. Coll. Surg. 46:427, 1973.

30. Rosenkrantz, Jens G.; Sullivan, Robert C.; Welch, Keasley; Miles, James S.; Sadler, Keith M.; and Paton, Bruce C.: Replantation of an infant's arm N. Engl. J. Med. 276:609–12, 1967.

CHAPTER 8

Tendon Injuries

ABSTRACT

Tendons must glide to and fro to carry out their function of transmitting force. Successful repair must restore continuity of the tendon without causing restrictive adhesions or joint stiffness. This problem is greatest in the flexor tunnels of the fingers where usually only one tendon should be restored, either by direct repair or tendon graft. The tunnel should be left open, except for small bridges, to allow pliable subcutaneous fat to surround the repair. Tendons should be repaired if the wound is clean and is seen early after injury, and if the risk of infection is small. All tendon surgery should be performed in the operating room. Technique should be atraumatic to avoid further injury. Incisions should be adequate and a bloodless field utilized. The steps of tendon repair and tendon graft are outlined as well as special techniques and postoperative care.

Pitfalls

1. Overlooked tendon lacerations
2. Overlooked associated injury, such as nerve and bone
3. Tendon laceration in flexor tunnel (No Man's Land)
4. Adhesions at site of repair
5. Infection
6. Joint stiffness

Three problems in the treatment of tendon injuries are:
1. Restoration of continuity
2. Prevention of adhesions
3. Prevention of joint stiffening

Tendons transmit force to joints from muscles located some distance away. Nature utilizes this mechanism to strengthen joint movement without creating bulk in the region of the joint to be moved. Methods of tendon union which take into consideration the large amounts of force involved are dealt with on the following pages, and these methods are usually successful. The prevention of adhesions is more difficult and leads to many failures. Adhesions about a tendon occur because of injury to the delicate gliding mechanism, and, unfortunately, this has already occurred by the

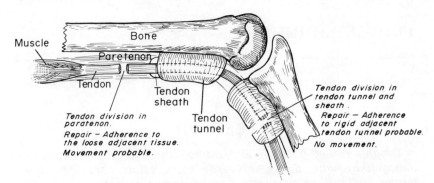

Figure 8–1. Tendon injury and repair in an area surrounded by paratenon or other loose, pliable tissue is much more apt to move after healing than a similar repair within a tendon tunnel.

time the patient is seen. However, it behooves the surgeon not to add to it.

The gliding surface of a tendon is either paratenon consisting of loose pliable tissue, when the tendon lies free and pulls straight, or a synovial sheath containing synovial fluid, when the tendon lies within a retaining tunnel and pulls around a corner, as in the volar aspect of the finger (see figure 8–1).

The success of a repair varies greatly in these two situations and will be discussed later in the section on zones of the flexor tendons. If adhesions occur to adjacent mobile tissue, such as paratenon, fat, or muscle, gliding movement will still occur, in contrast to adhesions in a fixed tunnel which prohibit normal movement.

The prevention of joint stiffening is largely a matter of maintaining movement and making periods of immobility as brief as possible. Recently, I have found periarticular injection of corticosteroids, such as triamcinolone acetonide, at the time of immobilization helpful to prevent stiffening. This is of special value when the period of immobilization must be prolonged or if there is injury about a joint.

PREVENTION OF FURTHER INJURY

To avoid further injury to the delicate structures of the hand during operation, the use of a bloodless field by means of a pneumatic cuff tourniquet is essential.

Every injury to the gliding surface of a tendon may lead to an adhesion. For this reason, it is also the duty of the surgeon to use the most delicate technique when working with tendons. Tendons should not be picked up with metal instruments except where the clamped portions of the tendons can be excised. The gloved fingers produce far less trauma than an instrument. A rubber drain, usually of a small size, placed about a tendon can be used to lift it from its bed and to label it while working with a group of tendons. A rubber drain is less traumatic than a cloth tape. Transfixation with a straight needle is a good method of manipulating the cut end of a tendon with minimal additional trauma. This and transfixation with a fine suture are both useful methods of controlling the free end of a tendon during repair (see figure 8–2).

INCISIONS

The wound caused by trauma is usually not ideal for exposure of the tendon nerve or vessel proximally and distally and should be supplemented to permit adequate exposure. Make extensions in the lines of Langer or parallel with skin creases whenever possible. Figure 8–3 summarizes by diagram some useful incisions of the wrist, palm, and fingers which heal with minimal scar.

Within the finger, special methods are necessary; incisions parallel to transverse folds do not give adequate exposure.

The Midlateral Incision

A midlateral incision gives good exposure of either the volar or dorsal aspects of the finger, depending on which flap is dissected free. The volar flap is usually dissected deep to the neurovascular bundles which are displaced with it. In this case, much care must be used in the region of the middle phalanx because the neurovascular bundle lies very close to the bone at this level and can readily be injured; the branches of the vessels and nerves to the dorsum of the finger will also need to be transected and ligated.

An alternative volar flap can be raised superficially to the neurovascular bundles. This flap has less vascularity than the former one but leaves the neurovascular bundles undisturbed. Although this alternative method has been advocated by English surgeons, I usually prefer the first method of lifting the neurovascular bundles with the volar flap, taking care not to injure them.

The Zigzag Incision

The zigzag incision, advocated by Bruner,[1, 2] gives excellent exposure of the volar portion of the finger and is particularly suited for tendon grafting and other volar surgery which requires postoperative immobilization. Additional dissection is necessary. The

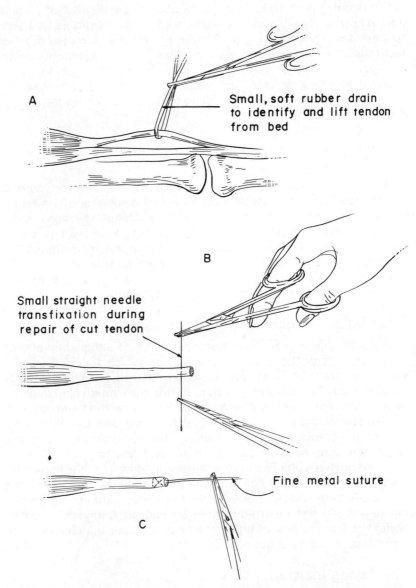

A

Small, soft rubber drain
to identify and lift tendon
from bed

B

Small straight needle
transfixation during
repair of cut tendon

Fine metal suture

C

Figure 8–2. Tendon manipulation. *A*, a small rubber drain causes little trauma when placed about a tendon. It identifies that particular tendon from others and allows it to be lifted from its bed with the least amount of injury. A fine straight needle *B* or a fine metal suture *C* are excellent methods of controlling a cut tendon so that it need not be picked up with metal instruments.

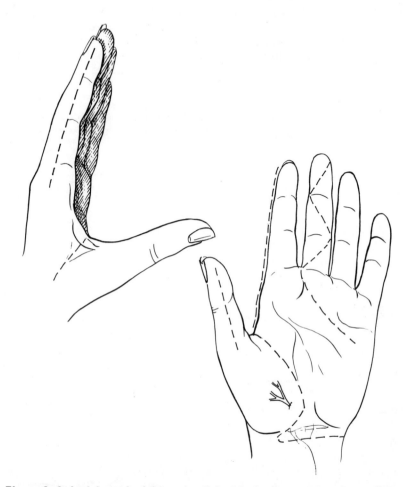

Figure 8–3. Incisions. Incisions parallel with the lines of Langer or flexion creases heal with the least amount of scar. In the finger, the midlateral incision gives good exposure. The zigzag incision gives excellent exposure, but is not recommended when early postoperative movement is to be employed.

distance between the volar joint creases of the finger does not change with flexion and extension. These creases must be crossed only at their lateral or medial ends. This incision gives good volar exposure, and the flaps heal well if they are left broadly attached at their bases.

I consider the zigzag incision inappropriate for tendolysis operations which are followed by early postoperative movement, but excellent for tendon grafting.

SUTURES FOR TENDON REPAIR

Tendons heal quite completely if their separated ends are approximated and held together for several weeks. It is not uncommon when reoperating months or even years later to be unable to recognize the site of a previous repair because of the complete reconstitution of a tendon.

Since healing is a slow process and the reaction about suture material itself causes an increased number of adhesions, a nonabsorbable inert substance is best. Silk, stainless steel wire, nylon,

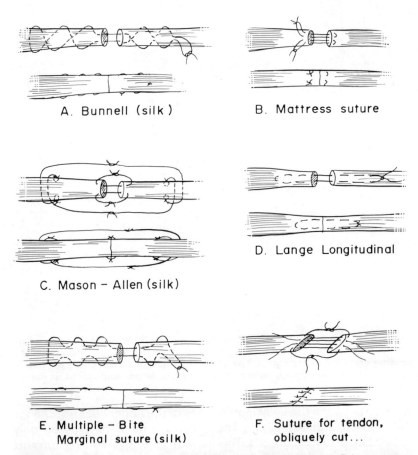

A. Bunnell (silk)

B. Mattress suture

C. Mason – Allen (silk)

D. Lange Longitudinal

E. Multiple – Bite Marginal suture (silk)

F. Suture for tendon, obliquely cut...

Figure 8–4. Various sutures for tendons. *A, B, C, D,* and *E* have secure purchase on the tendon fibrils and are recommended. *F,* simple stitches as illustrated here tend to pull free. (Redrawn, with permission, from Weckesser, Technique of tendon repair, in Injuries to tendons, chap. 8 of Flynn, J. Edward (ed.), *Hand Surgery* [Baltimore: Williams & Wilkins Co., 1966])

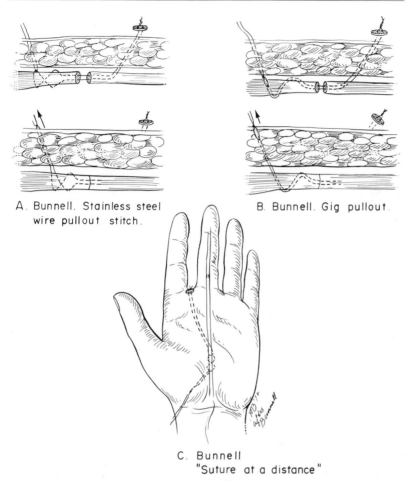

A. Bunnell. Stainless steel
wire pullout stitch.

B. Bunnell. Gig pullout.

C. Bunnell
"Suture at a distance"

Figure 8–5. Wire suture techniques. *A*, the Bunnell pullout technique. *B*, a simple gig pullout technique. In both *A* and *B*, the suture is removed completely in three or four weeks. *C*, is a method of removing muscle tension from the site of repair in the finger. (Redrawn, with permission, from Weckesser, Technique of tendon repair, in Injuries to tendons, chap. 8 of Flynn, J. Edward (ed.), *Hand Surgery* [Baltimore: Williams & Wilkins Co., 1966])

or some of the new plastic and plasticized materials meet these requirements best. The caliber of the material should be kept small.

For the types of tendon suture which have a "lateral purchase" on the longitudinal fibrils of the tendon, see figures 8–4 and 8–5.

A recent modification of the Mason-Allen stitch, which places more of the suture within tendon substance, is shown in figure 8–6.

Whenever adjacent pliable tissue is available, it should be brought in to cover the area of repair, thus preventing adherence to rigid

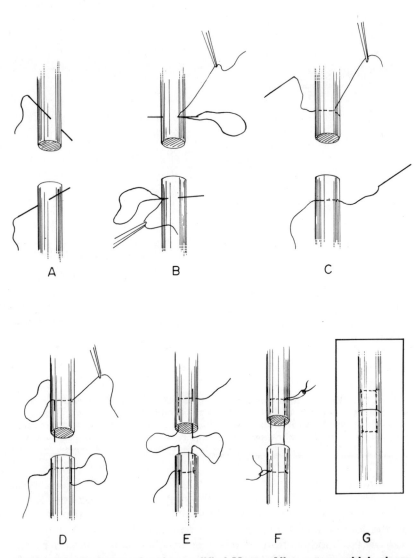

Figure 8–6. Technique for the modified Mason-Allen suture which places more suture within the tendon. (Redrawn, with permission, from Kessler and Nissim, Primary repair without immobilization of flexor tendon division within the digital sheath: An experimental and clinical study. Acta Orthop. Scand. 40:587–601, 1969)

nonmobile structures. Paratenon, fat, or muscle may be used for this purpose.

FLEXOR TENDONS

All things being equal, the results of flexor tendon repair vary greatly, depending on both the site of the injury and the probable development of restrictive adhesions postoperatively. For surgical purposes, the flexor surfaces of the fingers, palm, wrist, and forearm are divided into the zones shown in figure 8–7. Injury and repair within the flexor tendon sheaths, especially in Zone II, is the least likely to succeed owing to this tendency to adhere to the rigid walls of the tendon tunnels. Further complications occur because two flexor tendons are present in the Zone II tunnels. A decision whether to repair one or both tendons must be made. Usually only one tendon is chosen—the profundus.

Flexor Zone Tendon Repair

Table 8–1 is a summation of procedures considered most suitable under the various conditions of flexor tendon injury in the various locations. Zone I, the most distal flexor zone, contains only the distal joint flexor tendon (flexor profundus) and allows primary repair in the ideal case, especially in children, with a reasonable chance of success (see figure 8–8). If the division is at the distal or the midportion of the middle phalanx level, it can be repaired by advancement, making the distal insertion after the method of Wagner (figure 8–8C). If the case is severely contaminated or less than ideal for some other reason, cleansing, irrigation with sterile saline, and primary skin closure only are indicated. A tendon graft to the profundus about the intact sublimis can be done with less chance of infection later after the wounds have healed.

The most troublesome area, as mentioned, is the fibro-osseous flexor tunnel area (Zone II), the so-called No Man's Land of tendon repair. Here, if both tendons are divided, primary repair of only one tendon, the profundus, is usually advocated even if little trauma has occurred and the case is seen early after injury (ideal case). The strength of the sublimis unit is sacrificed for the sake of a greater chance of postoperative gliding motion of the profundus tendon alone (figure 8–9A and B). When the division is at the level of the p.i.p. joint, however—as listed under alternative procedures in table 8–1 and shown in figure 8–9C—one slip of the sublimis may be restored, but only laterally and away from the profundus repair.

TABLE 8–1
Flexor Zone Tendon Repair

Zone	Primary Treatment			Definitive Surgery	Alternative Procedures
	Most favorable Case seen early (4 to 6 hours after injury) Sharp laceration Minimal contamination Surgeon experienced	Less favorable Case seen late (6 to 12 hours after injury) Contamination Trauma Surgeon with limited experience	Least favorable Case seen very late	3 to 4 weeks after injury Wound well healed	
I Flexor profundus	Primary repair of profundus Advancement if necessary	Cleanse Debride Close skin		1. Secondary profundus repair advancement 2. Tendon graft through intact sublimis	Tenodesis of distal joint (not recommended)
II No Man's Land Both tendons divided	Primary repair of profundus *only*	Cleanse Debride Close skin	IN A L L Z O N E S — Treat for infection — Gain skin closure or coverage — Proceed with definitive surgery when wound well healed	Graft to profundus from palm to fingertip Excise divided sublimis	1. Reunite one slip of divided sublimis away from profundus repair (preferred in ideal cases) 2. Unite sublimis and profundus in proximal palm Transfer sublimis to finger in second stage[5] 3. Insert silastic implant Replace with graft 8 weeks later (Hunter technique)
III Thumb	Primary repair of flexor pollicis longus Advancement if necessary	Cleanse Debride Close skin		1. Delayed repair 2. Graft thumb (forearm to tip)	Secondary repair by advancement
IV Palm	Primary repair of all tendons and nerves	Cleanse Debride Close skin		Secondary repair of all tendons and nerves	
V Carpal tunnel	Primary repair of all tendons and nerves Leave carpal ligament open	Cleanse Debride Close skin		Secondary repair of all tendons and nerves Leave carpal ligament open	
VI Forearm	Primary repair of all tendons and nerves	Cleanse Debride Close skin		Secondary repair of all tendons and nerves	

IN ANY TYPE OF CASE DO NOT EXCISE AN INTACT SUBLIMIS

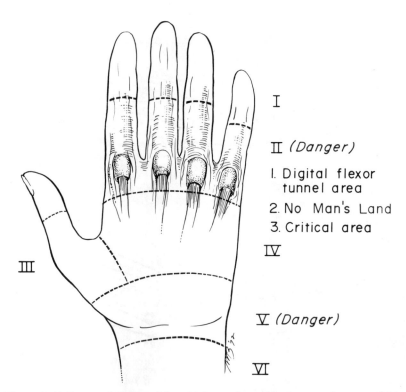

I

II *(Danger)*

1. Digital flexor tunnel area
2. No Man's Land
3. Critical area

IV

III

V *(Danger)*

VI

Figure 8–7. Zones of the hand in which results of tendon repair are variable. Poorest results are in Zone II (No Man's Land, the critical area). (Redrawn, with permission, from Weckesser, Technique of tendon repair, in Injuries to tendons, chap. 8 of Flynn, J. Edward (ed.), *Hand Surgery*, [Baltimore: Williams & Wilkins Co., 1966])

If conditions are less than ideal, no attempt at primary repair should be made in Zone II. The wound should be cleansed and closed and definitive surgery, consisting of a tendon graft, carried out three to four weeks later by someone versed in this type of work.

If the tendon tunnel has collapsed extensively at the time of tendon graft, a new pulley can be constructed as shown in figure 8–10.

Excision should be performed only when a sublimis tendon is divided in the No Man's Land area. An intact sublimis tendon should always be preserved. One slip of a divided sublimis tendon can be reunited in ideal cases, as mentioned.

Zone III, the flexor pollicis longus area of the thumb, contains only one flexor tendon but can still be the seat of troublesome adhesions. Adhesions here, however, do not interfere with function to the same extent as adhesions in Zone II. The excursion of the long flexor of the thumb is less than that of the long flexors of the fingers

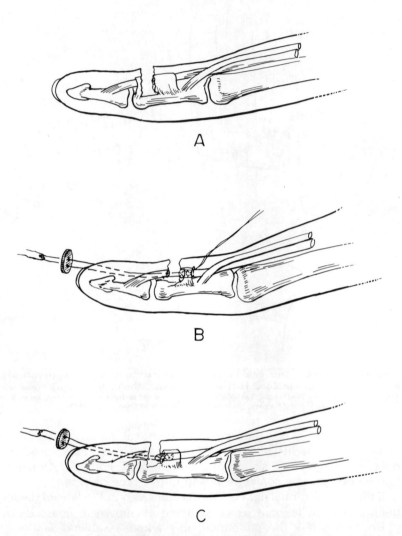

Figure 8–8. Flexor tendon repair. *A*, if the injury is clean cut and the patient is seen early, primary repair can be carried out, especially in children. *B*, the roof of the tendon tunnel is removed over the region of the repair to allow subcutaneous fat to surround the repair. *C*, from the middle of the middle phalanx distally, repair can be made by advancement. This places the repair further distal with less chance of adhesions. If the case is seen late or is dirty, the tendon repair should be delayed. Cleanse, debride, and close the wound or leave open with local antibiotic, as described under primary care in chapter 1. The suture shown is a pullout wire. This is optional, but the least reactive type of material should be utilized.

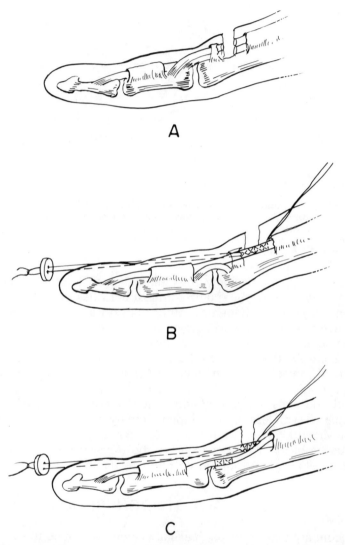

Figure 8–9. Flexor tendon repair in Zone II. *A,* cleanse wound, debride, and close skin. *B,* the tendon graft should be done at a later time except in ideal clean case which is seen early when primary repair of profundus tendon only is made. *C,* one slip of the sublimis may sometimes be repaired if this can be done away from the profundus tendon repair. The tunnel is unroofed over the area of the repair. Types of nonreactive suture are the option of the surgeon.

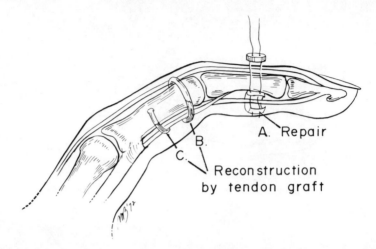

Figure 8–10. *A,* **repair of tendon pulley.** *B* **and** *C,* **methods of replacement of the tendon pulleys. These pulleys prevent bowing of the tendons on flexion of the digit.** (Redrawn, with permission, from Weckesser, Technique of tendon repair, in Injuries to tendons, chap. 8 to Flynn, J. Edward (ed.), *Hand Surgery* [Baltimore: Williams & Wilkins Co., 1966])

because the thumb has only one interphalangeal joint. In addition to this, the function of the thumb for most activities depends more on action opposite the fingertips rather than on extreme flexion. Lack of active flexion of the distal joint of the thumb does not cripple to the same extent as lack of active flexion of a finger.

In Zone IV, the palm, the flexor tendons have adjacent fat and lumbrical muscles which tend to prevent serious binding to adjacent rigid structures. This area is more like the forearm, Zone VI. In both these areas (Zone IV and Zone VI), tendons and nerves can be repaired with less risk of crippling adhesions. In the carpal tunnel (Zone V), structures are quite close together and adhesions can be a serious problem. It is best to leave the transverse carpal ligament open to allow more room in an effort to diminish adherence.

SECONDARY TENDON REPAIR

Secondary tendon repair is usually carried out three to six weeks after injury through a fresh incision after the wound has healed. This carries less chance of infection because it is done through a new sterile wound.

Unlike primary repair, the operator in secondary tendon repair may not have the advantage of normal joints with free movement unless special care has been taken. At the time of secondary repair, some stiffening may already have occurred.

No matter how good and how free the tendon repair is made, it cannot succeed if the joint it moves has stiffened. This is avoided by:

1. Preoperative passive movement to keep the joint capsule and ligaments supple. This requires special attention because the patient, being protective of the injured part, will tend to keep it at rest. Splinting should be avoided as much as possible for the same reason.
2. The local injection of corticosteroids into periarticular tissues. This is especially helpful during the postoperative period when joint immobilization must be carried out (see chapter 3, page 59).

EXTENSOR TENDONS

Exposure of extensor tendons is usually more readily carried out than exposure of flexor tendons. However, there exist specific problems centered around lessened excursion, thinner structure, weaker muscle pull, proximity to periosteum, and more complex anatomical arrangement.

In general, extensor tendons in traumatic wounds should be primarily repaired with nonabsorbable material after cleansing and debridement. But for wounds that are severely contaminated or seen more than six hours after injury, delayed repair is safer and there is less chance of infection. For these cases, close the skin only and allow primary healing of the injury. Definitive repair of the tendons can be carried out several weeks later through a fresh incision by someone versed in this type of work.

MALLET FINGER

The most distal injury commonly seen is avulsion of the extensor tendon from the base of the distal phalanx. The condition is sometimes referred to as "baseball" finger, but the causes are legion, and it may result from any sudden excessive force which tears the weak extensor tendon from its insertion, with or without a fragment of bone. The bent position of the distal joint resembles a mallet which has also led to the use of the term "mallet" finger (see figure 8–11).

If no bone is torn loose, splinting constantly for six weeks with the distal joint in extension and the middle joint of the finger flexed leads to union in the majority of cases. I prefer a well-padded cast which cannot be removed by the patient, but many splints have been devised which work if constantly kept in place.

If a bone fragment is torn loose, open operation is better. A stainless steel pullout wire about the fragment, tied over a button at the fingertip as shown in figure 8–11, can be used to give good reduction, but a padded cast is still recommended for six weeks. If a Kirschner wire is drilled across the distal joint to hold it in extension, care should be exercised not to place the joint in forced hyperextension because this shuts off blood supply and may lead to dorsal necrosis of soft tissues in the region expected to heal.

Flexion at the middle joint of the finger tends to advance the dorsal hood through the central slip insertion and to help close the gap over the distal joint.

Lacerations of the extensor hood over the middle phalanx beyond the central slip insertion may be treated in a manner similar to distal avulsion although a mattress suture of nonabsorbable material is more successful.

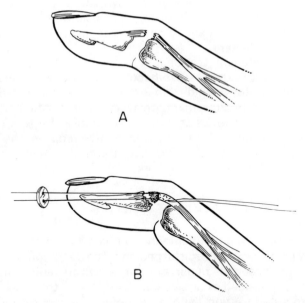

Figure 8–11. Mallet finger. *A,* the bent position of the distal joint of the finger when the extensor tendon is torn loose has led to the term "mallet finger" (other terms are "baseball finger" and "drop phalanget"). When the tendon is torn as shown in the diagram, immobilization for six weeks with the middle joint of the finger flexed and the distal joint extended is usually successful. *B,* if a bone fragment is torn loose with the tendon, replacement with a stainless steel pullout stitch is wise in addition to immobilization.

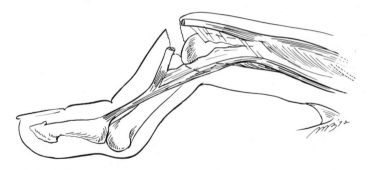

Figure 8–12. Boutonnière deformity. A tear or cut of the central slip of the extensor hood over the middle joint of the finger allows the joint to project dorsally through the cut tendon as through a "buttonhole." The lateral bands slip volarward and must be replaced dorsally when repair is carried out. Immediate repair of the central slip with dorsal replacement of the lateral bands gives best results.

ACUTE LACERATION OF THE CENTRAL SLIP (BOUTONNIÈRE DEFORMITY)

Acute division of the central portion of the extensor hood (central slip) near its attachment at the base of the middle phalanx allows the middle joint of the finger (p.i.p. joint) to fall into flexion (see figure 8–12). There is splitting and volar displacement of the lateral bands, as shown in the diagram. With this, the joint protrudes through the defect in the extensor tendon as through a buttonhole, giving rise to the name. The lateral bands being still intact pull the distal joint into hypertension. Flexion of the middle joint and hyperextension of the distal joint of the finger is frequently spoken of as boutenniere deformity, but it can also arise from the lateral bands being too tight after repair of mallet finger and from limitations of extension of the middle joint. In other words, it can arise from imbalance in the extensor hood or from middle joint stiffness. The most common cause is imbalance in the extensor hood, a result of laceration of the central slip.

Acute Repair

The best treatment of central slip lacerations is immediate suture with nonabsorbable material followed by four week's immobilization in extension. Care should be taken to replace the lateral bands of the extensor hood dorsally at the time of repair and to hold them there with fine sutures.

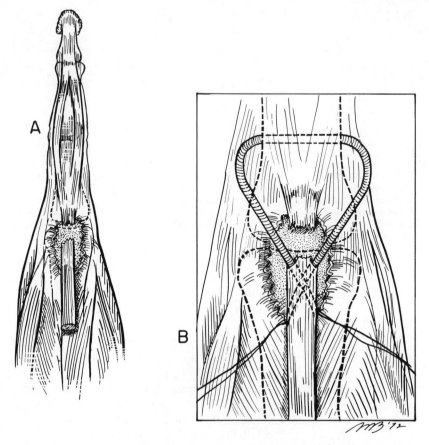

Figure 8–13. *A*, **late central slip laceration.** *B*, **repair by a crisscross tendon graft (Fowler). A tendon graft 3 mm in diameter is drawn through a drill hole in the proximal part of the middle phalanx, crisscrossed over the dorsum of the joint. It is sutured to the central slip proximally to overcome the slack in the central slip and to restore balance with the lateral bands.**

Late Repair

The following steps are recommended for late repair of central slip laceration:

1. If joints have stiffened, mobilize them prior to operation.
2. Carry out crisscross tendon graft (Fowler), as shown in figure 8–13.
3. Restore pull of lateral bands dorsal to center of rotation of middle joint.
4. Immobilize four weeks in extension.

LACERATION OVER PROXIMAL PHALANX, M-P JOINT, OR THE DORSUM OF HAND OR FOREARM

Injuries over the proximal phalanx, the M-P joint, or the dorsum of the hand or forearm require immediate repair with nonabsorbable sutures, followed by four week's immobilization in extension. Mattress sutures are suited to the flat, thin portions of the extensor hood. They should not penetrate the deep portion of the tendon in order to lessen the chance of adhesions to the periosteum. Woven sutures are stronger for the back of the hand and forearm where the risk of adhesions is less. The dorsal retinaculum over the wrist should be preserved except at the level of repair.

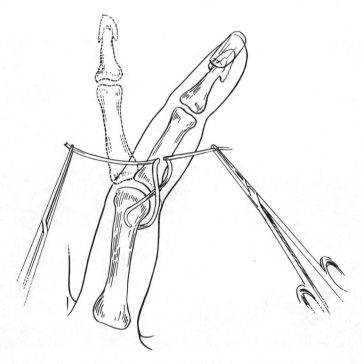

Figure 8–14. Volar ligament reconstruction. A portion of the palmaris longus (or other tendon) is threaded through drill holes placed volarward in the distal end of the proximal phalanx and the proximal end of the middle phalanx, as shown in this diagram. The graft is tightened after threading it double through one drill hole, and each end is then stitched to itself. The double threading is important to provide mechanical advantage for adequate tightening. It is tightened to hold the joint in *slight flexion*.

SWAN NECK DEFORMITY

Imbalance deformity with limited active distal joint extension, or swan neck deformity, occurs when the middle joint of the finger hyperextends. This is usually due to injury to its volar plate which also may be associated with disruption of the oblique retinacular ligaments of Landsmeer.

When the middle joint hyperextends, the lateral bands apply less extensor force to the distal joint, and it falls into flexion if the oblique retinacular ligament has been torn away. In some patients, removal of the sublimis tendon allows the middle joint to go into hyperextension. If Landsmeer's ligament is intact, however, its action will still allow the distal joint to extend, and the patient will manifest only "recurvatum" at the middle joint. I prefer ligament reconstruction, as shown in figure 8–14. The X ray of an illustrative case is shown in figure 8–15.

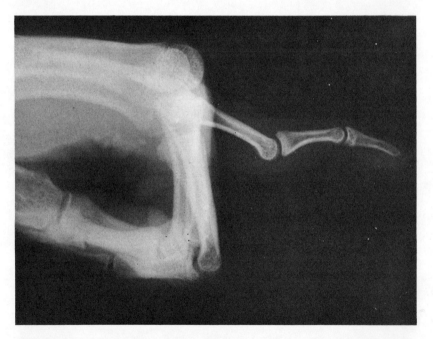

Figure 8–15. X ray of the right small finger of a 13-year-old girl struck by a football three years prior to appearing for treatment. The finger was severely hyperextended, tearing the volar capsule of the middle joint. Since that injury, when the middle joint hyperextended the distal joint had limited active extension, as shown. Her finger was awkward, and she bumped it frequently. Repair was accomplished through a volar ligament reconstruction.

This was repaired by a tendon graft placed between drill holes in the distal end of the proximal phalanx and the base of the middle phalanx, as shown in figure 8–14 (volar ligament reconstruction). The result was very satisfactory.

PRIMARY TENDON REPAIR

Whether or not, and when, tendon repair should be undertaken has been dealt with in previous paragraphs. If conditions are suitable, I proceed according to the following general outline:
1. Appropriate anesthesia
2. Pneumatic cuff tourniquet about upper arm
3. Skin and wound preparation to reduce bacterial contamination
4. Adequate skin incision (figure 8–3)
5. Identification and tagging of divided structures
6. Realignment of divided structures
7. Realignment and fixation of fractures (chapter 10), repair of tendons (figure 8–4), and repair of nerves, using magnification (chapter 9)
8. Skin closure or coverage
9. Splinting in relaxation
10. Elevation, antibiotics, specific immunizations

Anesthesia (see chapter 2), either general, supraclavicular brachial block, axillary block, wrist, or digital block, may be employed and is optional with the surgeon and the anesthetist. Intravenous lidocaine has become popular in recent years and is adequate for many procedures.

Tourniquet

The use of a pneumatic cuff tourniquet with a wide cuff inflated to between 250 and 300 mm Hg is essential to avoid further injury to delicate structures. It can be left in place for one and one-half hours without damage to a person with normal circulation (see chapter 1).

Skin and Wound Preparation for Surgery

Skin and wound preparation before surgery to reduce bacterial contamination should proceed in two stages (see figure 1–3, page 24).

Stage 1
   a. Skin of entire forearm and hand shaved
   b. Fingernails cleansed and trimmed short

   c. Surgical scrub (sterile gloves):
      soap or detergent
      brush and gauze
   d. Wound cleansed gently with detergent or soap
   e. Wound irrigated with one liter normal saline solution
Stage 2: change gloves and repeat 1 (*a* through *e*) with new setup.

Postoperative Care

At the close of the operation, stress is removed from the suture lines by placing proximal joints in a position of relaxation. This diminishes the pull across the suture line and minimizes the danger of postoperative separation. It is safest to allow the joints distal to the repair to have free movement in the direction of pull of the repaired tendon for the same reason (see figure 8–16).

Postoperative Immobilization

Immobilization should never be longer than necessary because of the danger of stiffening. In general, flexor tendons are immobilized three weeks and extensor tendons four weeks. Allowing the distal joints some movement, as shown in figure 8–16, also tends to diminish overall joint stiffening. This should be guarded active movement. Passive movements that do not place strain on the repair are valuable and should be utilized whenever possible.

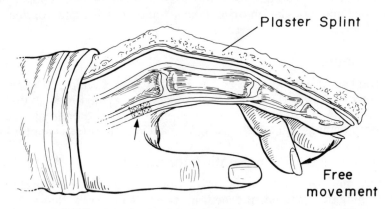

Figure 8–16. Postoperative immbolization. Less strain is exerted on the tendon repair if the joints distal to the repair (small arrow) are allowed to move in the line of tendon pull with protection against overextension (isotonic exercise).

The part is elevated postoperatively by bed sling to diminish edema. Postoperative antibiotics, such as penicillin G 300,000 units b.i.d., or suitable oral medication, such as erythromycin 250 mgm q.i.d., are given for four days except in very clean cases.

Infection can destroy the gliding mechanism and even produce necrosis of a tendon. It is the great enemy of successful tendon repair. Traumatic wounds should be gently cleansed with copious amounts of sterile saline solution as stated previously. For elective surgical procedures on tendons, the skin should be cleansed with detergent and the part enclosed in sterile material the night before operation. A careful preoperative skin preparation is also carried out at the time of surgery as well, and care is taken to diminish skin contamination during operation by keeping skin covered wherever possible.

The possible necessity for a tendon graft should always be discussed preoperatively with the patient and permission received to utilize graft if necessary.

TENDON GRAFTING

Tendon grafting is usually done as a secondary procedure, but is included here briefly for completeness, since it is the second-stage method of treatment of tendon injury.

Tendon grafts are utilized to replace a tendon which is missing or badly damaged. The graft in each case is completely detached from the donor area and is spliced into the recipient area where it regains new nourishment from tissue fluids and a new blood supply. Hopefully, this will occur with minimal lateral adhesion-formation. The danger of adhesions about a carefully placed graft is considered less than about most tendon repair areas. For this reason, grafts are utilized in the tunnel areas of the fingers (Zone II, No Man's Land). The distal union is made at the point of insertion at the base of the distal phalanx and proximal union, usually in the palm at the level of the lumbrical muscle. This places no sutures within the tendon tunnel. Preoperative care regarding joint mobility is the same as for secondary tendon repair. Great emphasis needs to be placed on having the joints freely mobile before tendon grafting since a post-operative period of splinting is a calculated risk during which some joint stiffening is bound to occur. A periarticular corticosteroid should be injected about the middle joint of the involved digit at the close of the operation to lessen problems with postoperative joint stiffness.

Preoperative skin preparation is the same as for delayed tendon repair. The use of the pneumatic cuff tourniquet is mandatory in my

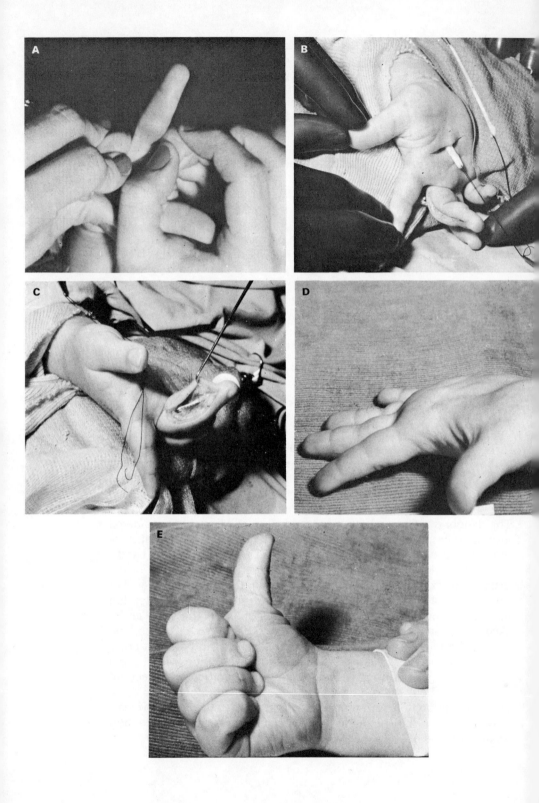

Figure 8–17. *A*, this two-year-old boy cut the volar surface of his right long finger on a bottle two months before this photo was made. There is no active flexion of the long finger although the joints are supple and the finger can be flexed passively into the palm. *B* and *C* were taken at the time of operation. The sublimis tendon, removed from palm to forearm and shown lying beside the child's hand in *B*, was placed as a graft from the palm to the tip of the finger. It was fixed distally into the stump of the old profundus tendon by means of a stainless steel pullout wire tied over a button, and in the palm by a silk "lateral purchase" suture. *D* and *E* show the result seven months later.

opinion. The anesthesia chosen should be effective in the involved extremity as well as in the tendon donor area.

Incision (figure 8–3) is made according to skin lines wherever possible. In the digit, the midlateral or volar zigzag incision is used. Recently I have been well pleased with the zigzag incision for tendon grafting because of the excellent exposure, especially at the base of the digit, although it does require more dissection. Healing has been quite satisfactory, with very little scarring.

Tendon grafting should proceed in this order:

1. Appropriate anesthesia
2. Pneumatic cuff tourniquet
3. Suitable skin incision:
    midlateral
    volar zigzag
    complementary palmar incision parallel with creases
4. Dissection and identification of divided tendon ends (secondary tendon repair suitable if gliding surface of tendon is well preserved and ends can be reapproximated without undue tension)
5. Tendon union by "lateral purchase" stitch
6. Mobile soft tissues brought into and around area of tendon union
7. Skin closure
8. Splint with tendon union relaxed and distal joints free to move in line of pull, as in figure 8–16 (postoperative immobilization approximately three weeks for flexor tendons and four weeks for most extensor tendons)
9. Systemic antibiotics for several days if dissection is prolonged or risk or infection increased for any reason

Figure 8–17 shows a two-year-old boy seen two months after a laceration on the volar aspect of the right long finger which healed promptly without treatment. No active flexion of the digit is seen in figure 8–17A.

At operation, the divided long flexor tendons were dissected free from the digit and palm through separate midlateral and palmar incisions. The sublimis tendon in this case was removed through a third transverse incision in the forearm and is seen lying beside the child's hand in figure 8–17B. This has been sutured into place in figure 8–17C by means of a stainless steel pullout wire tied over a button at the distal union and a silk repair in the proximal palm. He wore a cast for four weeks postoperatively with the wrist in flexion to diminish the pull on the repair. The result seven months after repair is seen in figure 8–17D and E.

The tendon unions were kept out of the tunnel area by means of the graft. The distal one was beyond the distal joint in the area of normal insertion of the tendon and the proximal one in the palm at the level of the lumbrical muscle origin.

This technique by experienced operators can yield good results in a high percentage of cases if the scarring is not severe. If the scarring is severe, the special technique of Hunter and Salisbury[4] is probably a wiser one to use. Sources of tendons for grafting are shown in figure 8–18.

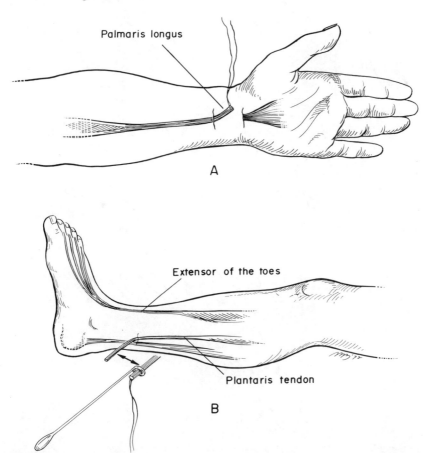

Figure 8–18. Sources of tendon grafts. Any fresh, noninjured tendon of somewhat smaller size than the original can be used. The sublimis tendon can be used as a flexor tendon graft although it may be a little large in some cases. *A* shows the palmaris longus tendon (not present in about one-fifth of the people), and *B* shows the plantaris tendon on the medio-anterior aspect of the Achilles tendon. If the plantaris tendon is not present, an extensor of the second, third, or fourth toe may be used.

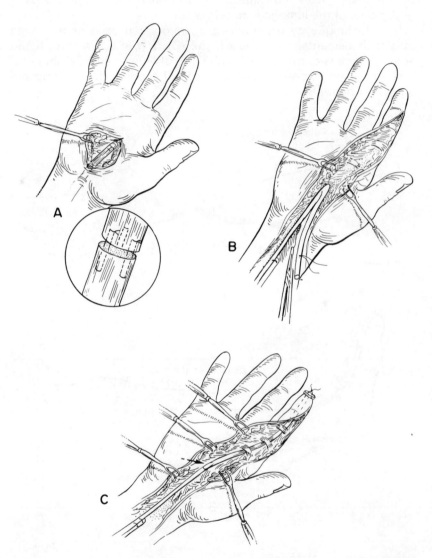

Figure 8–19. Paneva-Holevich two-stage tenoplasty. *A*, primary stage.
The sublimis and profundus tendons are united at the level of the lumbrical
muscle. *B* and *C*, the second stage is carried out one month later. The
sublimis tendon is detached from its muscle belly in the forearm and turned
distally as an extension of the profundus tendon to the base of the distal
phalanx. Early motion (sixth day) is utilized. (Redrawn, with permission, from
Paneva-Holevich, Two-stage tenoplasty in injury of the flexor tendons of the hand. J. Bone Joint
Surgery 51-A: 21–32, 1969)

TWO-STAGE SUBLIMIS TENDON REVERSAL
(PANEVA-HOLEVICH)

The two-stage sublimis tendon reversal technique developed by Paneva-Holevich[7] (figure 8–19) involves uniting the sublimis and profundus tendons in the proximal palm at the time the original wound is debrided. The original wounds are closed and allowed to heal.

Three to six weeks later, reoperation is carried out. The involved sublimis tendon is dissected free from its muscle belly in the forearm and turned distally, as an extension of the profundus to its original insertion at the base of the distal phalanx. As a result of the previous union in the base of the palm, only one repair (at the distal insertion) is required at the second stage. This allows earlier postoperative movement. The union in the palm tends to be bulky and must be kept in the proximal palm where there is room for it to move. Limited experience with this technique has been favorable.

THE HUNTER ARTIFICIAL TENDON TECHNIQUE
(STAGED FLEXOR TENDON RECONSTRUCTION)

James Hunter[3, 4, 5] of Philadelphia has done much recently in developing an artificial tendon made of dacron and silastic.* The dacron in its center gives strength and prevents sutures from pulling out. The external silastic prevents reaction within the tissues. "It serves as an inert, flexible, non-adhering implant to bridge areas of scar tissue with gliding motion while a new mesothelial-like sheath develops in injured areas around the surface of the implant. . . . Undamaged tendon sheath is preserved and linked with newly formed tendon sheath so that a soft gliding bed is established."[3]

Early in his work, Hunter, as others, attempted to permanently replace damaged tendon with artificial tendon but gave this up. He now advocates it only as a mold across scarred areas about which a new synovial sheath forms. It is his opinion that movement of the prosthesis in its bed leads to a better sheath formation. This is accomplished by passive movement of the digit. The technique now advocated is for "less than ideal cases." It is carried out in two stages.

At the first stage, the prosthesis is inserted from the distal insertion of the finger to the distal forearm after excision of any severely scarred tendon or sheath. At the second stage, carried out about four months later, a tendon graft is pulled into the new tunnel as

---

* Available from Extracorporeal Medical Specialties, Inc., Royal and Ross Roads, King of Prussia, Pennsylvania 19406.

the prosthesis is removed. This tendon graft, placed through the previously formed mesothelial-lined tunnel, is then inserted distally and motored by an appropriate muscle, usually in the distal forearm.

Results to date have been encouraging. The technique is recommended for cases which have more than the usual amount of scar tissue. It is not considered necessary in favorable cases when little scarring is found. Extra care must be exercised regarding aseptic technique since infection is a calamity requiring removal of the prothesis.

COMBINED USE OF PANEVA-HOLEVICH AND HUNTER TECHNIQUES

In the late repair of a severely scarred tendon in the finger the combination of these two techniques is logical. The author has used them together with success and they have been reported upon favorably by Chong, Cramer and Culf.[9]

In this combination technique used during reconstruction, the silastic rod is placed to the level of the lumbrical muscle in the palm and at the same time, a union is made between sublimus and profundus tendons at that level.

At a subsequent stage, about three months later, the sublimus tendon is detached from its muscle belly and threaded distally as the silastic rod is removed.

With only a distal tendon union present careful active finger flexion is begun the day after surgery with a dorsal protective cast in place as shown in figure 8–16.

REHABILITATION

The period of immobilization must be followed by a closely supervised period of active mobilization. The joint changes from the immobilization are more readily reversible the sooner postoperative motion is started. Patients vary greatly in their ability to follow instructions and to move postoperatively stiffened joints which give pain on movement. The services of a skilled physical therapist are very helpful here, but the surgeon continues to have responsibility and should work closely with the therapist during this critical period of rehabilitation if best results are to be obtained. It is the surgeon's responsibility to have the patient regain active movement. The use of the voluntary muscles of the extremity requires conscious effort, and this must be encouraged and directed by the surgeon and the

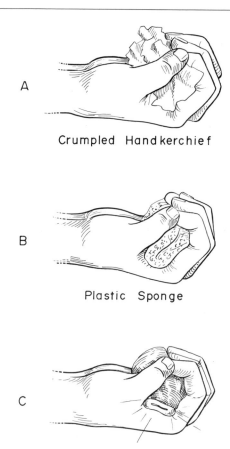

A

Crumpled Handkerchief

B

Plastic Sponge

C

Bulb with Air Vent

Figure 8–20. Exercise to regain movement. Objects to grip are conducive to active movement. They should allow nearly complete flexion. The air bulb with an air vent (C) is excellent. Minimal dressings are also conducive to movement.

therapist. In contrast to involuntary muscle function, voluntary function does not return spontaneously. Most patients must be urged to use their extremity after operation; some will use it too much and this must be guarded against also.

Frequent observation by the surgeon as well as the therapist is the best and safest way to keep the patient progressing. Occupational therapy is also helpful, especially for those who do not have a specific hand activity to which they can return. Close cooperation between the physical therapist and the patient should be encouraged. The surgeon should encourage occupational efforts as soon as healing has proceeded to the point where force can be safely transmitted over the repaired tendon. This must be carried out gradually. Active flexion and extension without resistance is encouraged after the third or fourth week, and resistance is started gradually ten to fourteen days later. Figure 8–20 shows some of the soft objects which may be used in the palm in the early postoperative period. The object must be collapsible so that flexion is complete.

Hot-water soaks to the hand and forearm twenty to thirty minutes t.i.d. are a great help at home. A mild soap that will suds and cleanse the skin is a pleasant addition which patients appreciate.

The increase in flexibility provided by the heat of the soaks is considered desirable in spite of the increase in local tissue fluid which is produced. Elevation and exercise can be used to diminish the latter.

Bibliography

1. Bruner, Julian M.: Optimum skin incisions for the surgical relief of stenosing tenosynovitis in the hand, Plast. Reconstr. Surg. 38:197–201, 1966.
2. Bruner, Julian M.: The zig-zag volar-digital incision for flexor-tendon surgery, Plast. Reconstr. Surg. 40:571–74, 1967.
3. Hunter, James M.: Artifical tendons: Early development and application, Am. J. Surg. 109:325–38, 1965.
4. Hunter, James M., and Salisbury, Roger E.: Use of gliding artificial implants to produce tendon sheaths: Techniques and results in children, Plast. Reconstr. Surg. 45:564–72, 1970.
5. Hunter, James M., and Salisbury, Roger E.: Flexor-tendon reconstruction in severely damaged hands: A two-stage procedure using a silicone-dacron reinforced gliding prosthesis prior to tendon grafting, J. Bone Joint Surg. 53-A:829–58, 1971.
6. Kessler, Isidor, and Nissim, Fuad: Primary repair without immobilization of flexor tendon division within the digital sheath: An experimental and clinical study, Acta Orthop. Scand. 40:587–601, 1969.
7. Paneva-Holevich, E.: Two-stage tenoplasty in injury of the flexor tendons of the hand, J. Bone Joint Surg. 51-A:21–32, 1969.
8. Weckesser, Elden C.: Technique of tendon repair, in Injuries to Tendons, pp. 186, 187, 191, 192, chap. 8 of Flynn, J. Edward (ed.): *Hand Surgery* (Baltimore: Williams & Wilkins Co., 1966).
9. Chong, J. Kenneth; Cramer, Lester M.; and Culf, Norris K.:

Combined Two-Stage Tenoplasty with Silicone Rods for Multiple Flexor Tendon Injuries in "No Mans Land," J. Trauma 12:104–21, 1972.

CHAPTER 9

Nerve Injuries

ABSTRACT

The nervous system depends upon functionally intact neurons to transmit sensory, motor, and sympathetic impulses. Function may be interrupted with the nerve still grossly intact, indicating conservative treatment. However, the surgeon is usually required to repair nerves which have been completely divided. Nerve injury should be recognized at first examination by sensory, motor, and pseudomotor testing.

The controversy between early and late repair is giving way to primary repair in clean cases seen early after injury, if experienced personnel are available. Meticulous repair is possible with the use of head loupe magnification for debridement and the microscope for the repair proper.

Pitfalls

1. *Unrecognized nerve division*
2. *Unrecognized associated injury*
3. *Infection*
4. *Joint stiffness*
5. *Neuroma formation*

The nervous system, the communicative portion of living tissue, carries out its function through the prolongation of specialized cytoplasm—axons—which transmit directly through cell substance, in contrast to hormonal communication which is mediated by substances carried in the bloodstream to other distant cells. The nervous system offers quick instantaneous communication to and from specific parts of the anatomy like a telephone system, while the hormonal system is more like the mails, taking longer but affecting receptors in many parts of the body.

The nervous system supplies one of the main methods by which contact is made with the environment and by which one part of the anatomy keeps in touch with another part, coordinating body function, internal and external. Impulses from the external environment (picked up from or near the external surface)—somatic sensations—are dealt with at a conscious level, where decisions are made regarding the body's position and location and the proper alterations for overall well-being and safety.

156

Impulses concerned with internal function of the body, largely dealt with at a subconscious level, are mostly reflex or automatic. These regulatory, automatic or sympathetic nervous system impulses consist of sensory and motor elements also but, unlike the external sensory, there is little or no way of testing internal sensory elements. Peripheral sensory elements of many types—touch, heat, pain, and so forth—transmit impulses centrally to the brain, and each of these can be tested in case of injury. The peripheral motor impulses activate muscle while sympathetic impulses control glandular function and probably carry out many other coordinating functions about which very little is known at present. In the extremities, the peripheral nerves are groupings of axons that transmit impulses centrally and peripherally for both the somatic and the sympathetic system. Some are purely sensory and others purely motor, but most contain both types of axons. The sympathetic fibers in peripheral nerves are best known for their pseudomotor and peripheral vascular tone, and it is these parameters which can most readily be tested to determine whether a particular nerve is intact. This aspect is especially valuable when voluntary cooperation is lacking, as in children and certain adults. This is referred to later under methods of testing nerve function.

ETIOLOGY OF NERVE INJURIES

Nerve injuries can be classified as follows:
1. Physiological interruption:
      contusion
      compression
      moderate ischemia
      alterations of metabolism (such as diabetes)
      moderate temperature changes
2. Physical interruption:
      laceration
      severe contusion
      electrical injury
      severe ischemia
      severe heat or cold (burns; freezing)
      chemical damage

Nerve continuity can be interrupted by any of these mechanisms. The interruptions may be physiological with preservation of gross continuity, or, more frequently, there may be complete physical separation.

According to the observations of Waller, made more than one hundred years ago, the axon and myelin below the site of transection injury become fragmented and are absorbed over a period of several weeks, the endoneurial tubes being emptied out in preparation for the regrowth peripherally of the new axons. Schwann cell and macrophage activity are intense during this period of wallerian degeneration.

The Peripheral Axon

Figure 9–1 is a diagram of myelinated peripheral axon showing the relationship of the myelin, the Schwann cell, and the endoneurium. The segment between successive nodes of Ranvier is occupied by one Schwann cell. Injury, if severe enough to divide an axon, leads to degeneration peripherally (wallerian degeneration) and proximally to the next node of Ranvier or at least to the nucleus

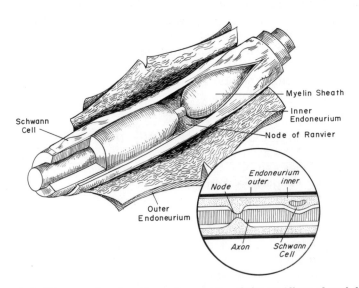

Figure 9–1. Diagram showing the various parts of the myelinated peripheral nerve fiber. (Redrawn, with permission, from Sunderland, *Nerves and Nerve Injuries* [London: E. & S. Livingstone, 1968])

of the nearest Schwann cell. The latter appears to take part in the mobilization of enzymes and phagocytes which clear out the endoneurial tube in preparation for the peripheral extension of a new sprouting axon, which ideally enters before local fibroblastic activity interferes. Flows of axoplasm within the axon have been recognized and efforts to assess the function of these in relationship to nerve repair following injury are being made.

Nerve injury has been classified into seven degrees by Sunderland.[3]
1. First degree:
>interruption of conductivity at site of injury
>anatomical continuity preserved
>no wallerian degeneration (neurapraxia of Seddon)
2. Second degree:
>axons severed
>failure of axon to survive below level of injury
>endoneurium and balance of nerve trunk preserved
3. Third degree:
>more severe trauma
>any or all of first and second degree injury, plus disorganization
>of internal structure of funiculi
>destruction of endoneurial tube continuity
4. Fourth degree:
>more severe disorganization with much tangling of connective
>tissue, Schwann cells, and axons
>nerve trunk grossly in continuity
5. Fifth degree:
>loss of continuity of nerve trunk
6. Partial and mixed lesions:
>damage different to different parts of nerve
7. Irritative lesions:
>late manifestations
>abnormal motor and sensory phenomena

In clinical work, differentiation is made only between continuity and severance of the traumatized nerve trunk (first and fifth degrees). However, the amount of injury to the intact nerve trunk (second, third, or fourth degree) is significant in determining the degree of recovery which is possible. An attempt should be made to estimate the degree of trauma to the intact nerve as well as the degree of trauma to the divided ends of the nerve trunk, and in the latter case, the severed ends of the nerve should be cut back to the untraumatized nerve as much as possible, within limits which still allow restoration of continuity. Fourth degree injuries possibly should be resected, but in practice few surgeons have done this, thinking that the grossly traumatized architecture of the intact nerve will transmit new axons better than a suture line.

Figure 9–2 shows a digital nerve traumatized by a power drill. The patient had complete anesthesia along the radial border of the tip of the finger after injury. Surgical exposure, as shown in this photograph, demonstrated that the nerve was physically intact. Recovery of sensation occurred spontaneously several weeks after injury, indicating a first degree injury. Anesthetic agents applied next to a nerve trunk also prevent the conduction of impulses temporarily; this is a physiological type of interruption, in effect similar to first degree injury caused by trauma, although the length of interruption is shorter.

Physical interruption caused by trauma is the type of nerve injury

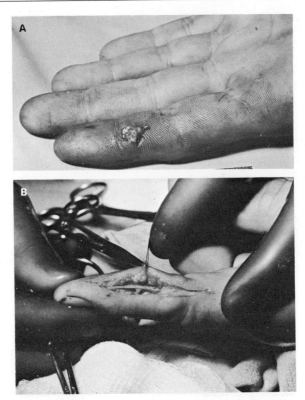

Figure 9–2. Traumatized digital nerve. *A,* this young man penetrated his left index finger with a power drill while at work. He had anesthesia distal to the point of entrance of the drill. *B,* operation showed the nerve was grossly intact. Sensation returned spontaneously.

most often encountered by the surgeon and the one which most often offers the greatest challenge. The problem here is one of restoring the continuity of the axons of the nerve, or better, reconstituting the gross architecture of the nerve so that the axons can regrow to the periphery.

TESTING FOR NERVE FUNCTION

The determination of loss of nerve function is of first importance as soon as possible after injury, because it signifies the degree of seriousness of the injury and assures proper treatment at the earliest possible time. Tests should be made in the emergency room or at the time the case is first seen. They can be carried out quickly with the following plan.

1. Conscious sensory
   a. Check median, ulnar, and radial nerves for:
      pinprick
      2-point
      touch
2. Conscious motor
   a. Check median nerve for contraction of opponens muscle
   b. Check ulnar nerve for contraction of first dorsal interosseous
3. Subconscious sympathetic
   a. Check median, ulnar, and radial nerves for:
      pseudomotor (sweating)
      ninhydrin test
      starch-iodine test
      temperature change with block

Both sensory and motor tests as well as those for sympathetic function, when indicated, should be carried out distal to the site of injury. Tendon function tests should also be carried out because of the frequency with which tendons and nerves are injured simultaneously With experience, these tests can all be done quickly.

The sensory tests of touch, pinprick, and 2-point should each be carried out in the region of the three major nerves to the hand using the instruments shown in figure 1-1, page 19.

1. Median: thumb, index, and long fingertips
2. Ulnar: small finger
3. Radial: dorsal cleft (thumb and index finger)

The motor tests are made on muscles distal to the site of injury. For practical purposes the intrinsic muscles of the hand are readily available, can be easily tested, and represent the terminal motor connections of the median and ulnar nerves. The radial nerve is sensory only beyond the wrist.

Figure 1-2 (page 20) shows palpation of the opponens muscle of the thumb for median nerve function and the first dorsal interosseous muscle for ulnar nerve function. These muscles can be felt to tighten beneath the fingertips, making this an objective test for the examiner, and they can both be tested simultaneously if the patient pinches his thumb and index fingertips together firmly. Palpating contraction of an intrinsic muscle, another objective test, is less subject to error.

Sympathetic function, not being under voluntary control, is also objective. It can frequently be observed by watching for beads of perspiration on the fingertips when the pinprick test is carried out. Positive sweating in any peripheral nerve area indicates that the nerve is intact in that area since the sympathetic fibers to sweat glands and blood vessels travel in the main peripheral nerves. The ninhydrin and starch tests are refined ways of recognizing the presence of perspiration in the area supplied by any nerve. Their usefulness is limited by the need for special reagents and materials. The tests are especially useful, however, in children and in adults when exaggeration or malingering is suspected (see page 21, chapter 1).

NERVE REPAIR

The surgeon does not have control over the extent of the original injury but should recognize its degree before proceeding with nerve repair. The trauma to the divided nerve ends dictates the amount of disorganization present. A blunt, tearing force injures much more than a sharp, cutting force. A saw injury is hence different from a knife injury. The amount of contamination varies with the location of the accident. A street injury differs from a kitchen injury in that more contamination occurs and the hazard of infection is thus greater.

PRIMARY OR DELAYED NERVE REPAIR

There has been controversy about when to repair a severed nerve. Some controversy still remains.

The factors favoring early repair are:
1. The nerve and adjacent structures are usually more readily identifiable.
2. Retraction has not occurred.
3. Fibrosis is not as great.
4. Morbidity is less.
5. Joint stiffness is less.

The factors favoring late repair are:
1. Elective procedure can be planned when all facilities are available and optimal.
2. Necessary personnel can be assured.
3. Danger of infection is less.
4. Limit of injury is more readily identifiable.
5. Patient is aware of extent of injury.

No hard and fast rule can be given to insure the right decision to this problem. Certainly the danger of infection is one of the greatest deterrents to carrying out definitive repair in a fresh wound. Infection is less when the wound is a sharp one and is seen early after injury.

War wounds and gunshot wounds are different from the sharp clean wounds seen in civilian life. When factors of personnel and facilities are equal, it is my opinion that a clean, sharply divided nerve, seen early, should have its continuity restored at the earliest possible time. This view has been supported by the work of Grabb,[2] who found a higher grade of motor reinnervation of the intrinsic muscles of the hand in monkeys following primary repair of sharply divided median and ulnar nerves at the wrist.

NERVE REPAIR TECHNIQUE

The greatest service of a surgeon is to restore the divided nerve as accurately as possible with as little additional injury as possible at the earliest time that this can be done safely. For a sharply severed, clean injury this can be done at once, as just described. If conditions are less than ideal, the wound should be debrided and the skin closed; definitive repairs can be carried out four to six weeks later through a fresh incision.

Recently, delayed primary repair has been practiced with success. The wound is irrigated and cleansed and covered with an antibiotic solution, such as 0.5% neomycin solution or some other broad spectrum drug, for four to six hours when delay is necessary for any reason. An injured child with a full stomach may be treated in this way (see chapter 1). Absence of suitable operative personnel or operative space are other good reasons for choosing this procedure.

Accurate apposition of the nerve ends can be done best under magnification. An attempt should be made to realign funiculi and to suture them when feasible. The realignment of funiculi is complicated by the rapidly changing arrangement of these structures along the course of a peripheral nerve. Sunderland[3] points out that the pattern of funiculi is altered so rapidly that transverse sections of a nerve taken even more than a few millimeters apart are different.

Grabb et al.[2] have attempted to identify funiculi by electrical stimulation in order to make more accurate nerve anastomoses. In a comparison of methods of peripheral nerve suture in monkeys, they concluded that funicular nerve repair gave better results but that identification of funiculi by size and position was more practical.

In actual practice, nerve injuries are frequently associated with skin, tendon, muscle, and joint injury. Often, broad areas and large wounds are involved. How to use the magnification of the operative microscope with its very limited field in such a large wound can be a frustrating problem. A method of nerve repair, which I prefer, utilizes the ocular loupe as well as the microscope for different stages of repair.

1. Ocular loupe with ×2–3 magnification.
   Repair associated injuries.
   Debride nerve ends.
   Realign nerve ends.
   Stay sutures to epineurium.
2. Operative microscope with ×10–16 magnification:
   Recheck funicular alignment.
   Attempt funicular suture if feasible (limitations).
   Repair epineurium.

Value of Nerve Repair

Regeneration after nerve repair is variable even when the best techniques are employed. In general, the younger the patient and the more peripheral the lesion, the better the results. It is a universal observation that recovery is best in children; the reasons for this have not been elucidated. The more peripheral the lesion, the more isolated are the motor and sensory elements, so that sensory axons are more apt to be restored to sense end organs, and motor fibers to muscle, if alignment is good. Also, within sensory and motor elements, the more peripheral the repair, the less reorientation is required centrally to restore proper function.

Figure 9–3 shows the forearm of a seven-year-old girl whose arm was virtually amputated, except for the radial artery, in an automobile accident. The bones were fixed and the muscles of the forearm restored on the day of injury. The median and ulnar nerves were sutured in the mid-forearm seven weeks later. She has regained quite good sensation in her left hand. Intrinsic motor function has returned. She has good use of her hand. It is very doubtful that an adult would have had such successful return of function. However, partial return of function is very valuable and makes peripheral nerve repair very worthwhile at any age, if the restored sensation is not painful.

RESTORATION OF SENSATION BY ISLAND PEDICLE TRANSFER

The island pedicle (see chapter 4) can be utilized to restore sensation to an important tactile area. This is a method of transferring intact sensation and vasculature.

Figure 9–4 shows the partial amputation of the index finger in a thirty-seven-year-old workman. Length of the digit was partially maintained by means of an abdominal pedicle flap. In order to give acute sensation in opposition with the thumb, the border of the ring finger, with its intact nerve and blood vessels, was transferred as

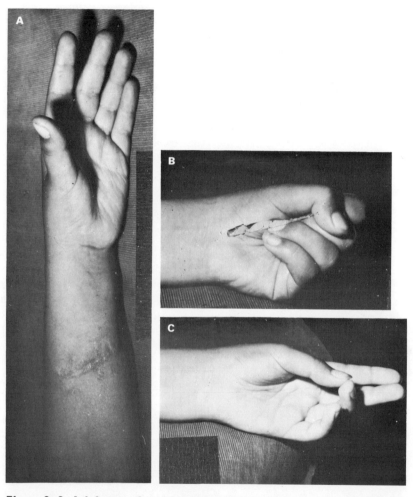

Figure 9–3. *A*, left arm of a seven-year-old girl which was virtually severed in its distal third except for the radial artery. Bone and muscle continuity was reestablished on the day of injury by George Bertino, M. D., and the median and ulnar nerves were repaired seven weeks later. *B* and *C* show an excellent return of intrinsic and extrinsic muscle function. She has 4 mm 2-point sensation in her digits.

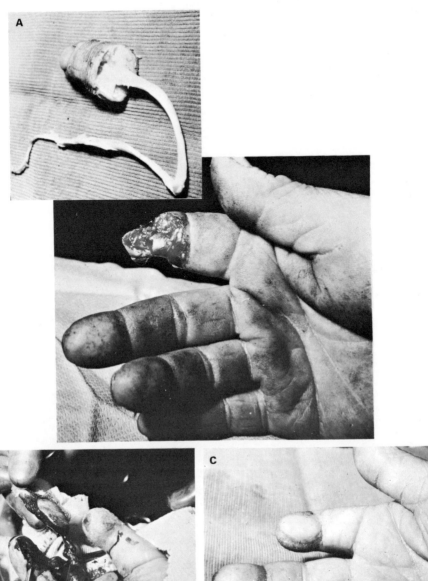

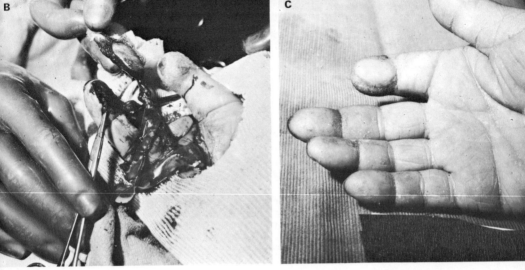

Figure 9—4. *A*, the right index finger of a thirty-seven-year-old man which was caught in a lathe, tearing off the end of it (*inset*) and avulsing the flexor tendon as shown. A primary abdominal pedicle flap was utilized to preserve the length of the protruding phalanx. *B*, an island pedicle flap with its own blood vessels and digital nerve is being elevated from the ring finger and transferred to the pedicle flap extension of the index finger to give epicritic sensation. *C*, this is a very effective way of providing normal sensation to an important tactile area.

shown in figure 9–4*B* and *C*. He gradually became accustomed to the border of his ring finger being on the index finger.

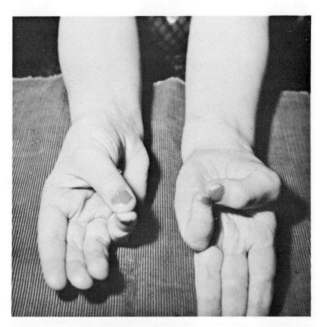

Figure 9–5. This six-year-old girl lacerated her left wrist on a storm door four months earlier. Median nerve and flexor sublimis tendon of the ring finger were lacerated. Both were repaired on the day of injury. Note her inability to oppose the thumb to the small finger in a normal manner as seen in the right hand because of paralysis of the opponens muscle. The function of the hand is greatly reduced by this inability to bring the thumb opposite the fingers. Four months after this photo she has good opponens function and good sensation and was using her hand normally.

UNREGENERATED MOTOR NERVE INJURY

The following are examples of unregenerated motor nerve injury which show characteristic changes in the hand. The changes in posture and shape result from denervation of the intrinsic muscles supplied by each nerve. Figure 9–5 is an acute injury which showed recovery four months later. Figures 9–6 through 9–8 are cases seen late after injury for which tendon transfer was the only available method of regaining function. By this technique, a less important movement is sacrificed to restore function by substitution.

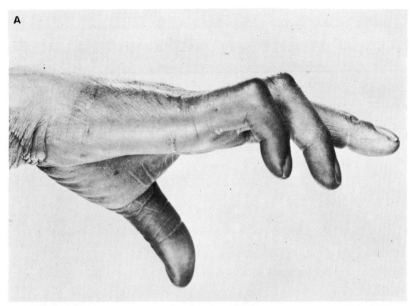

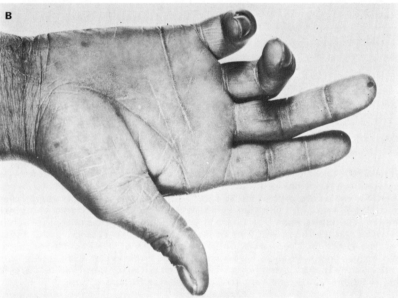

Figure 9–6. A wound of the forearm sustained several years earlier in which this man's ulnar nerve was injured. No repair had been carried out. He had obtained some sensory return over the small and ring fingers, but paralysis of the interosseous and lumbrical muscles to these digits had resulted in this typical claw deformity of his ring and small fingers. (The interosseous and lumbrical muscles are the primary flexors of the M-P joints.) His index and long fingers, however, are not clawed because the remaining lumbrical muscles are innervated by the median nerve.

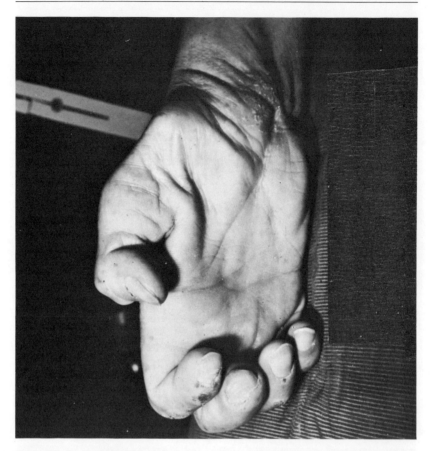

Figure 9–7. Complete claw hand in a forty-nine-year-old man. No intrinsic muscles are functioning. All interossei, the thenar muscles, and the hypothenar muscles are paralyzed. At age 17 the volar aspect of his right wrist was blown away in a shotgun accident destroying both median and ulnar nerves. The digits were nearly anesthetic and only the extrinsic (forearm) muscles and tendons were functioning. There was no balance in the digits for fine function. There were no primary flexors of the M-P finger joints and no opponens or abductor of the thumb. Function of the fingers was improved by plantaris tendon graft between extensor carpi radialis brevis and extensor hoods, and ring sublimis transfer for opposition.

Figure 9–8. A and B, complete claw hand except for the abductor digiti quinti in an eighteen-year-old man, who sustained a brachial plexus injury fourteen months earlier from a rifle bullet wound of the left pectoral region which also injured his brachial artery. C and D, M-P joint flexion was restored by transfer of ring and long finger sublimis tendons to the extensor hoods (sublimis transfer), and the abductor of the small finger was transferred across the palm to give opposition to the thumb.

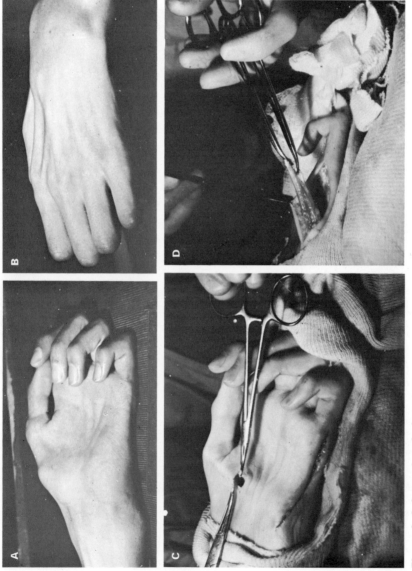

Figure 9–8. Legend on facing page.

Bibliography

1. Grabb, William C.: Median and ulnar nerve suture: An experimental study comparing primary and secondary repair in monkeys, J. Bone Joint Surg. 50-A: 964–72, 1968.
2. Grabb, William C.; Bement, Spencer L.: Koepke, George H.: and Green, Robert A.: Comparison of methods of peripheral nerve suturing in monkeys, Plast. Reconstr. Surg. 46: 31–38, 1970.
3. Sunderland, Sydney: *Nerves and Nerve Injuries*, pp. 2, 26, 127 (London: E. & S. Livingstone, 1968).

CHAPTER 10

Injuries to Bones and Joints (Fractures of the Hand as Related to Function)

ABSTRACT

Fractures of the phalanges and metacarpals require the same basic principles of treatment as broken bones in other parts of the body, plus greater attention to accurate reduction of the fracture and to the care of joint soft tissue. This is due to the smaller size of the structures and the necessity to maintain mobility in the many small joints of the hand. The small joints are very subject to stiffening from immobilization, and, for this reason, immobilization should be kept at a minimum and internal fixation utilized freely to restore movement at the earliest possible time. Rotational deformity in the phalanges and metacarpals may not be readily visible in an X ray and is best avoided by observing and treating the fingers in flexion so that the digits fit comfortably together during grasp.

Wrist movement is compound, occuring not only at the radio-carpal joint but between most of the intercarpal joints as well. The midcarpal joint between the lunate-triquetrum bones and the multangulars (the capitate-hamate bones) is spanned by the carpal navicular bone, which is thus subject to frequent injury. In forced dorsiflexion of the hand, the navicular bone may fracture if this force continues, and dislocation dorsally of the distal carpus may occur (perilunate dislocation), or the lunate bone may dislocate volarly.

Reduction is usually readily carried out by traction on the fingers. Any of the carpal bones may be fractured by the various forces to which they are subjected at times. Joint surface disruption should be reduced as accurately as possible, as in the phalanges and meta-carpals. Since fractures of the navicular are subject to a great deal of movement during motion of the wrist, these fractures should be treated by wrist immobilization in plaster until healed radio-graphically.

Pitfalls

1. Failure to make an X ray examination

173

2. *Failure to recognize an unstable fracture*
3. *Joint stiffness because of immobilization*
4. *Incomplete reduction of joint surface*
5. *Malunion*
6. *Immobilization with finger straight*
7. *Rotational deformity with overlapping fingers (not recognized during straight-finger immobilization)*
8. *Dependence upon X ray appearance to determine rotational reduction*
9. *Failure to repair ligaments when dislocated finger does not reduce with a sharp "snap"*
10. *Overlooked navicular fracture*
11. *Overlooked lunate dislocation*

Cases in Which the Outcome Is Apt to Be Less Than Desirable — Early Referral Advisable

1. *Unstable fracture of phalanx of metacarpal*
2. *Fracture involving a joint surface*
3. *Displaced or comminuted fracture of proximal or middle phalanx*
4. *A dislocated joint which does not reduce with a "snap" (torn collateral ligaments)*

Bone, one of the hardest and the most widespread of the firm tissues of the body, offers rigidity and support. In addition to holding the body up against gravity and helping to maintain its shape, the bones make possible the system of levers and pulleys (joints and tendons) by which the voluntary muscles give purposeful movement.

The structural stability of the small bones of the hand and the mobility of the joints between them make possible the dexterous movements on which most hand function is based. Fine, nimble movement, strengthened by the large muscles of the forearm, along with extremely acute sensation represent the most important forms of hand function. These functions the surgeon should make every effort to maintain and restore.

The surgeon should remember that injury producing a fracture of a bone also produces tearing and hemorrhaging in adjacent soft tissues which may be less obvious but as deleterious to future function as the fracture itself.

The multiple digits of the hand and the multiple joints in each digit provide adaptability which makes possible the wide range of function of the hand. Such a multiple-part structure allows some compensation for loss of function following injury, but in view of the wide functional requirements of the human hand, it is important that normal function be restored as completely as possible to each part.

The small size of the fifteen bones and the fifteen joints of the digits does not diminish their value or simplify their treatment. A digit that is stiff or does not move properly in relationship to the other digits can be a severe crippling influence in the hand. The small size in itself complicates treatment. More accurate reductions of fractures are necessary in order to preserve movement and to keep that movement in the proper plane so that motion of adjacent digits is properly complemented rather than hindered. Teamwork between digits is normally an important part of hand function, and this requires the agility and precision of each digit.

The basic principles of treatment of fractures of the hand are essentially the same as for the treatment of fractures in other parts of the body except for certain additional features which take into account the factors just discussed. Treatment of hand fractures should be as follows:

1. Reduce accurately.
2. Immobilize.
3. Prevent joint stiffening (see page 59, chapter 3).

The most important factor in the prevention of joint stiffness is movement. Most people can overcome the stiffening which occurs in the small joints as a result of immobilization for up to two or three weeks. Beyond this time interval, there is great danger of permanent impairment. Continued, active to-and-fro movement is the best method of overcoming early joint stiffness. Gentle passive assistance is of great value and can usually be best applied or supervised by a physical therapist. The surgeon can play a very great role at this point along with the physical therapist by making repeated measurements and offering encouragement to the often-bewildered or discouraged patient.

COMPLICATIONS OF HAND FRACTURES AND DISLOCATIONS

The complications of fractures and dislocations in the hand must be considered:

1. Joint stiffness
2. Malunion
3. Loss of structural rigidity:
   nonunion of fractures
   ligament disruption
4. Adherence of adjacent tendons

Since accurate reduction of fractures and the preservation and early restoration of joint movement are so important in maintaining function of the hand, open reduction and internal fixation are frequently indicated in order to regain movement at an earlier time.

TREATMENT

In carrying out the principles just discussed and in providing the quickest restoration of normal hand function, the first observation to make regarding a fractured bone in the hand is whether or not the fracture is stable (see figure 10–1). If the fracture is reduced, will the fragments remain together or will they tend to become displaced once again?

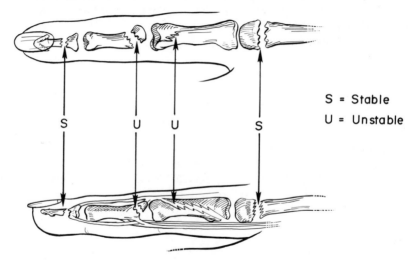

S = Stable

U = Unstable

Figure 10–1. In any fracture of a phalanx or metacarpal, the examiner must decide whether it is stable or whether it enters a joint surface. Unstable fractures are usually best treated by internal fixation. Those entering a joint surface require especially accurate reduction and, frequently, internal fixation.

The second thing to determine is the condition of the joint surfaces. If the fracture is an unstable one which would tend to slip out of place either by the pull of adjacent tendon insertions or the overall collapsing force of more distally inserted tendons, or if the fragment is large and causes a significant disruption of an articular surface, open operation should be carried out in order to gain accurate reduction and firm internal fixation. If the fracture is transverse so

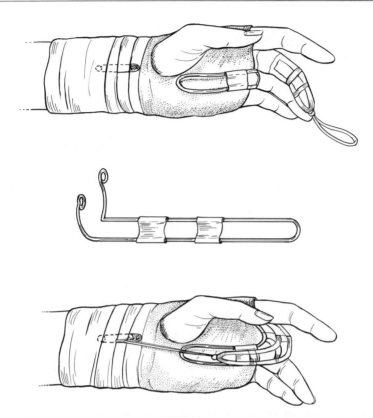

Figure 10–2. Method of external fixation of stable fractures of phalanx or metacarpal after reduction. Follow-up X rays should be made at the end of the first week, at least. After two weeks the finger can be freed periodically to carefully exercise the immobilized joints.

that the fragments impinge quite securely on one another, immobilization by external fixation (figure 10–2) will probably be adequate. But it is wise to X-ray the position at the end of the first week to be sure that no displacement has occured. If it has, restorative measures are still possible.

Internal fixation can usually be accomplished by Kirschner wires drilled either longitudinally through the phalanx or metacarpal, or at angles across the fracture line. Their placement is best made with a power drill so that attention can be focused on direction of insertion of the Kirschner wire and on maintenance of accurate reduction of the fracture during the insertion. Open operation is preferred. It is probably best to cut the Kirschner wires so that they retract just beneath

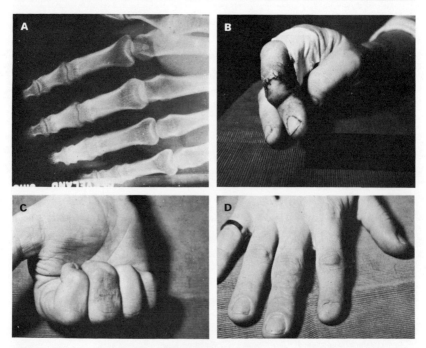

Figure 10–3. *A*, X ray of an index finger which was caught in a hamburger patty press. The finger had been amputated at the base of the nail through the distal phalanx and the phalanx projected beyond the soft tissues. *B*, the amputated tip of the finger has been covered by a flap from the adjacent long finger to give soft tissue padding over the exposed phalanx. *C* and *D*, result of the operative procedure ten months later.

the skin but are still palpable and can be readily located when time for removal occurs four to six weeks later. If they are allowed to project through the skin, special care should be taken to prevent infection by keeping the areas dry or by the application of an antibiotic ointment periodically to the areas of skin penetration.

Exposure for fracture reduction of phalanges is usually best through midlateral incisions of the digit. Traumatic wounds often do not give adequate exposure, and the surgeon should not be hampered by this. Transverse incisions on the dorsum of the hand which parallel skin creases are usually adequate for exposure and reduction of metacarpal fractures. The four metacarpals of the fingers offer a special anatomical situation in which a broken metacarpal can be quite adequately splinted by Kirschner wires drilled transversely into an adjacent intact metacarpal. Usually two, and sometimes three, wires are required to give good immobilization. Longitudinal Kirschner wires are also quite effective for immobilization, and especially so when multiple metacarpals are fractured.

FRACTURE OF THE DISTAL PHALANX

The most distal bone in the finger is most frequently subjected to trauma. Fractures of the tuft usually heal satisfactorily with simple immobilization. However, nonunion can be a problem near the base of the phalanx; the instability of an un-united fracture of the distal phalanx of the index finger recently required a bone graft in a doctor who used his index finger to pipet solutions in his laboratory.

Transection of the end of a finger through the distal phalanx (as shown in figure 10–3) is a common occurrence which offers specific problems in repair if the length of the digit is to be properly preserved. The solution, by means of a cross-finger flap, is shown in *B*, and the result nine months later, in figure 10–3*C* and *D*. Good function of the finger without sacrificing length was restored by this means. (See the section on fingertip injuries, chapter 7, for a more complete discussion of this problem and for alternative methods of treatment.)

Avulsion at an epiphysis is demonstrated by the child's X ray shown in figure 10–4. This four-and-one-half-year-old boy caught the end of his long finger in a folding chair as he sat down. The

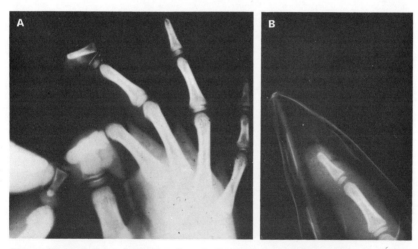

Figure 10–4. Epiphysis dislocation. *A*, X ray of the right hand of a four-and-a-half-year-old child who caught his long finger in a folding chair as he sat down, causing a dislocation of the epiphysis. The dislocation was reduced, *B*, and immobilized for four weeks. Healing was complete, and further growth has occurred. The diaphyseal cartilage plate was not broken.

dislocation occurred transversely through the junction of the diaphyseal cartilage plate and the diaphysis (Type I epiphyseal fracture[1]). This was replaced under digital block anesthesia by dorsal pressure. It returned to its normal location without difficulty and was splinted in straight position for four weeks. Growth was not interrupted because the cartilage plate was not broken.

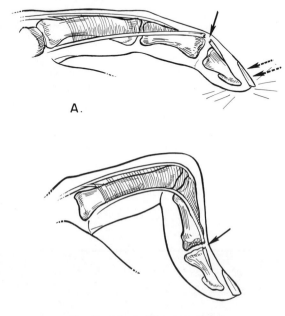

A.

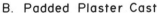

B. Padded Plaster Cast

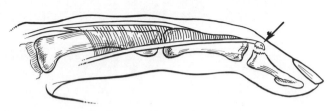

C. Open Operation

Figure 10–5. Mallet finger. *A*, this condition results when a sudden excessive force is applied to the tip of the finger, either tearing the tendon or pulling loose a fragment of bone. *B*, the tendon tear is treated by immobilization for six weeks in the position shown. *C*, if a bone fragment is torn loose, open operation and repair with a stainless steel pullout wire is indicated.

MALLET FINGER

Mallet finger may be associated with an avulsion fracture of the base of the distal phalanx, as shown in figure 10−5. X rays should always be made to determine its presence. This is an unstable fracture because of the pull of the extensor tendon. If there is avulsion, I recommend open reduction with a pullout wire tied over a button before applying a padded plaster cast for six weeks. The cast alone is recommended in those cases with avulsion of the tendon insertion without fracture (see page 137, chapter 8).

AVULSION OF THE
FLEXOR PROFUNDUS TENDON

Avulsion of the flexor profundus tendon is also a possibility, although it is less frequent than avulsion of the extensor tendon. It must be repaired surgically at the earliest possible time after injury to restore flexion of the distal joint of the finger.

The flexor profundus may tear loose from its insertion with or

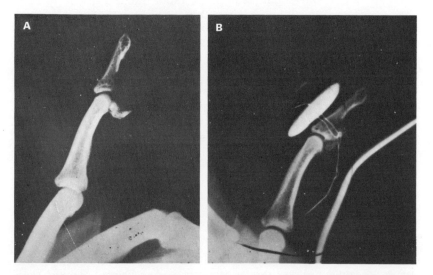

Figure 10−6. *A*, Avulsion of flexor profundus tendon by forceful flexion of the distal joint of the finger while wrestling. Immediate repair by open operation is mandatory whether or not a bone fragment is torn away. *B*, replacement by Bunnell pullout wire and button. The button shown is larger than necessary. Beware of this injury. It produces no deformity, and can be recognized only by detecting lack of active flexion.

without a bone fragment, just as the extensor tendon, but with the distinction that this type of case always requires open operation because of retraction of the flexor tendon (see page 132, chapter 8).

Figure 10–6 shows the X ray of a young patient who was not able to flex the distal joint of the long finger after wrestling with a friend. This, of course, is an unstable fracture. Immediate repair is necessary in this type of case to restore function. Replacement by Bunnell pullout wire is shown in the postoperative X ray (figure 10–6B). This type of repair works well whether or not a bone fragment is present and is recommended immediately after injury in both types of avulsion. Motion can be started after two weeks. The pullout wire is removed at the end of four weeks.

FRACTURES OF THE MIDDLE PHALANX

The middle phalanx has the sublimis tendon attached to its base on the volar aspect, which acts as a strong displacing force for fractures in that vicinity. In addition to this, the overall collapsing forces of the more distally inserted flexor profundus and extensor hood tend to produce overriding of unstable fractures.

Figure 10–7 shows an oblique unstable fracture in the middle phalanx of the small finger of a thirteen-year-old boy who had broken his finger while starting a lawn mower six weeks earlier. With the amount of overriding shown in the photograph, flexion would never be possible at the distal joint. At open operation, through two midlateral incisions, alignment was restored as shown in figure 10–7 B and C. At present, adherence of the extensor tendon over the associated proximal phalangeal fracture is still limiting movement of the middle joint, and he is receiving active and passive physical therapy exercises. His ability to use his hand continues to improve, and he has the chance of further improvement with the alignment now present.

Figure 10–8 shows the X ray of a twenty-eight-year-old man struck on the end of the right long finger with a baseball two days previously during an outing. The patient had much pain and swelling

Figure 10–7. _A_, X ray of the middle phalanx of a thirteen-year-old boy's right small finger, the seat of an unstable overriding fracture of six weeks' duration. Distal joint flexion was impossible. _B_, the method of fixation after open reduction. _C_, appearance after removal of the Kirschner wires three months later. Motion is still limited because of adherence of the extensor tendon over the proximal phalanx but may be benefited by tendolysis and early motion.

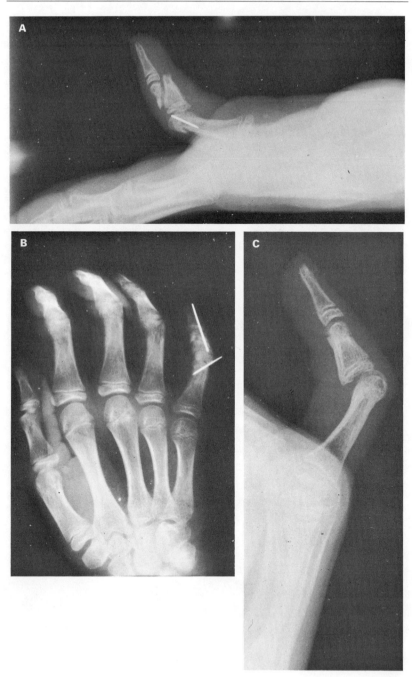

Figure 10–7. Legend on facing page.

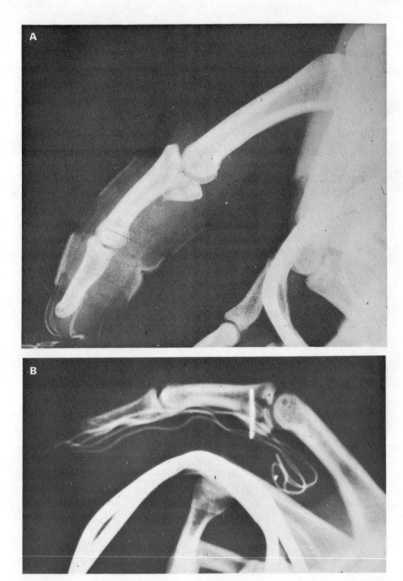

Figure 10–8. *A*, a fracture altering the joint surface which resulted from a baseball striking the tip of the finger. *B*, reduction was by open operation. Painless movement of the joint is present fifteen years later.

of his finger. Because of the joint surface alteration, open reduction was carried out through a midlateral incision and the fragments fixed with a Kirschner wire, as shown in figure 10–8 *B*. The splint was removed and motion started on the tenth day after operation. He now has a complete range of painless movement fifteen years after injury.

Figure 10–9 shows transection of the base of the middle phalanx and central slip of the extensor hood in a band saw while cutting meat. The fracture was immediately reduced and fixed (figure 10–9 *B*). Active movement was started carefully at twenty-one days and gradually increased. The movement present six months later is shown in figure 10–9 *C* and *D*. It is felt that the internal fixation which allowed early movement was an important factor in the successful treatment of this patient.

Figure 10–10 shows X rays of the right hand of a forty-six-year-old man after it was caught in a press. The middle phalanges of the index, long, and ring fingers are seen to be severely comminuted. The soft tissues of the end of the long finger were nonviable, requiring amputation through the middle phalanx. Rather than amputating these three fingers through their middle joints, the unstable fragments of bone were reduced and pinned together with Kirschner wires. The fractures of the index finger were stable and were held on a volar plaster splint, as shown in figure 10–10*B*, for three weeks. Motion was then started with the hope of maintaining middle joint mobility of the fingers. This is probably the best that can be done in such a severe case.

DISLOCATION OF THE PROXIMAL INTERPHALANGEAL JOINT

Just as excessive force applied to the shaft of a bone may lead to fracture, excessive force applied to a joint may lead to dislocation. Sometimes both occur simultaneously, and for this reason X rays should be made whenever either is suspected. Dislocation of the joint surfaces of two bones may occur by stretching and partial tearing of the capsule and collateral ligaments or the ligaments may give way completely. The state of the ligaments must be evaluated clinically because they do not cast a shadow on the X ray. The suddenness with which reduction occurs and the stability of the joint once it has been reduced give the necessary information. If the joint reduces with a sudden "snap" when traction is applied, this is an indication that the collateral ligaments are still intact. This is further verified if the joint is stable and remains intact when

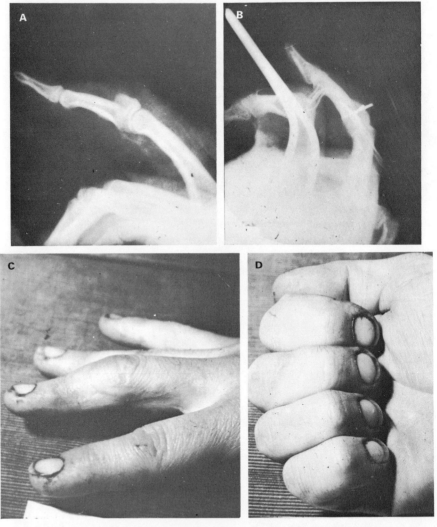

Figure 10–9. *A*, X ray of the right hand of a thirty-year-old man who cut his long finger on a band saw transecting the base of the middle phalanx and the central slip of the extensor hood. *B*, the fragment has been reduced and immobilized with Kirschner wires. The central slip of the tendon was repaired with black silk. *C* and *D* show the range of movement six months after repair.

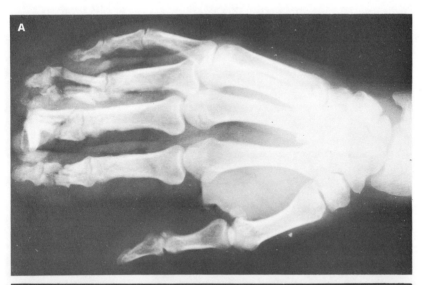

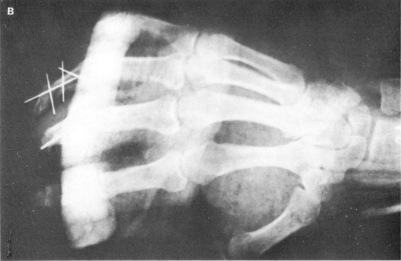

Figure 10–10. *A*, X ray of the right hand following a press injury. The distal tissues of the long finger were nonviable because of extreme compression and had to be amputated through the middle phalanx. The comminuted fragments of the ring finger were reduced and held with Kirschner wires. *B*, the postoperative X ray. Healing occurred and the fingers were preserved, though joint stiffening limited return of function.

movement is carried out following reduction. Active motion of the joint should be started about one week after injury to preserve mobility.

Figure 10–11 shows the X ray of a fifty-year-old woman who twisted her right long finger in a fall. It is seen that the middle phalanx lies volarward and is angulated ulnarward. First treatment consisted of digital block anesthesia and longitudinal traction. When this was carried out, the finger straightened into normal aligment,

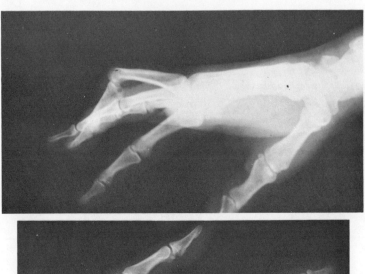

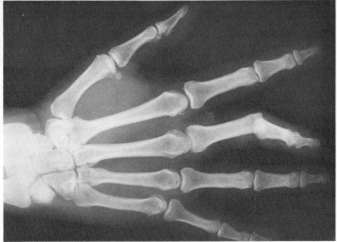

Figure 10–11. X rays of a fifty-year-old woman's right hand taken after a fall in which her long finger was twisted and displaced as shown. Under anesthesia the finger could be pulled into a straight position but no sudden "snap" occurred, indicating a torn collateral ligament. The dislocation reoccurred when traction was reduced. The radial collateral ligament and the central slip of the extensor hood were then repaired at open operation.

but *no sudden snap occurred during reduction*. When motion was carried out following reduction, recurrent dislocation occurred. With these two observations as a guide, the patient was admitted to the hospital and the joint was explored through a radial midlateral incision of the finger. The radial collateral ligament was found completely disorganized and the central slip of the extensor hood also disrupted, with the joint herniating through it to form a boutonnière deformity. Both tendons were repaired with silk, and the finger was splinted to allow healing to get underway. Active motion was begun at three weeks to prevent severe joint stiffness. Twenty months after repair, the patient had active extension of the middle joint to 20° of a straight line and flexion to 90°. The joint was stable and useful, though slight boutonnière deformity of the finger persisted. The finger was very useful to her. If the immediate repair had not been done, secondary operation would have been necessary with the result less satisfactory, in my opinion.

FRACTURES OF THE PROXIMAL PHALANX

Although there are no large tendon insertions to the proximal phalanges, the collapsing force of more distally inserted tendons is even greater here than for the middle phalanges. Hence, there is a great tendency for displacement to occur. Also, the risk of the flexor or extensor tendon or both becoming caught in the callus of bone repair is greater here than over the middle phalanx. If this occurs, motion of both interphalangeal joints is restricted and the result is poor. Secondary tendolysis followed by early movement may be successful in such cases, and should be attempted. At present, the only way to prevent tendons from becoming caught in callus is movement during the period of fracture immobilization, and, of course, this may lead to displacement of the fracture unless it is quite stable or is internally fixed.

Figure 10–12 shows the X ray of a forty-year-old man who had caught his right hand in a machine a few hours earlier. There was a compound fracture dislocation of the middle joint of the right finger with the bone protruding. The wound was cleansed and explored in the operating room soon after injury. The volar capsule of the joint was repaired with silk. The fracture reduced readily and was stable after being re-placed. In view of its mobility, no internal fixation was utilized, and active movement was started two weeks after injury by periodically releasing the finger from its splint, as shown in figure 10–2.

Figure 10–13*A* shows the X ray of a seventeen-year-old factory worker who had caught his left ring finger in a tow motor five

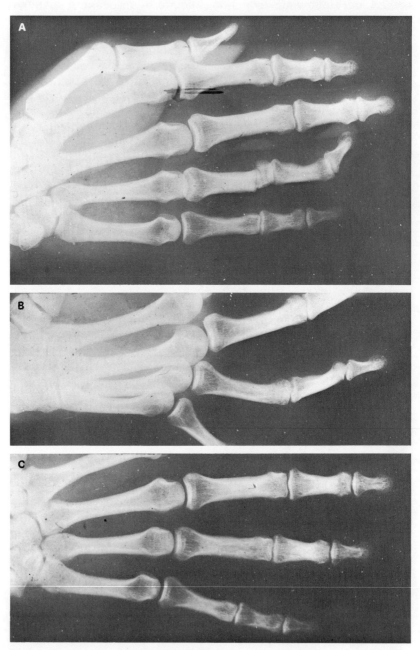

Figure 10–12. Legend on facing page.

weeks earlier. The finger had been treated on a straight splint and no follow-up X ray made until just prior to his referral. It is seen that the position of the fragments is unsatisfactory. There is 25° movement present in the middle joint. Flexion is blocked by the proximal fragment. Figure 10–13*B* shows the method of internal fixation utilized. Active movement was started on the fourteenth postoperative day. The follow-up appearance by X ray is also shown in figure 10–13*C* and *D*. Follow-up photographs taken two and a half years later, figure 10–13*E* and *F*, show firm flexion against the palm with 60° flexion at the middle joint. This is less than normal but is very useful movement, enabling him to use his hand quite well, which would have been very unlikely with the position of the fragments that existed when first seen.

BENNETT'S FRACTURE (FRACTURE OF THE HOOK OF FIRST METACARPAL)

The normal function of the thumb involves free movement to and from a position opposite the fingers. The pulp-to-pulp apposition thus provided greatly enhances the function of each finger. This movement of the thumb is caused by the participation of both the intrinsic and extrinsic muscles, but it is especially provided by the thenar muscles. It also depends upon free movement at the carpometacarpal joint which, in turn, depends upon the normal hook shape of the proximal end of the first metacarpal bone. This saddle joint cannot function normally and thumb motion is greatly impaired if the normal relationships at the proximal end of the first metacarpal are not restored.

Forces applied to the tip of the thumb are borne largely by the hook of the first metacarpal at its base, and, hence, fractures are frequent. When this occurs, the base of the first metacarpal rides proximally and radially, and the hook usually stays in the "saddle" over the greater multangular. The fracture is very unstable. At the same time it is readily reduced by distal traction on the thumb. Constant elastic pull with a Kirschner wire through the shaft of the

Figure 10–12. *A,* **X ray of a forty-year-old man's right hand which had been caught in a machine a short time earlier. There was a compound fracture dislocation of the middle joint with bone protruding. Open reduction was carried out in the operating room after meticulous cleansing. The volar capsule was repaired. No internal fixation was used for the fracture because it was stable after reduction. Active movement was started two weeks later by temporarily releasing the finger from its splint.** *B* **and** *C,* **show the X ray appearance one year later.**

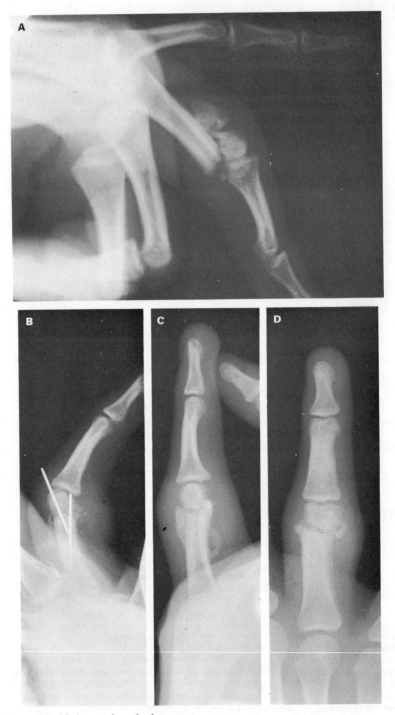

Figure 10–13. Legend on facing page.

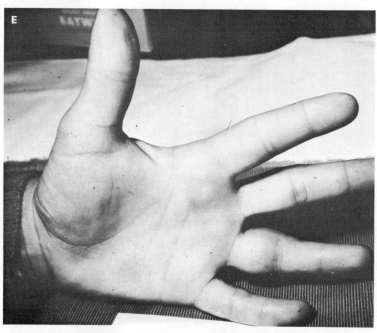

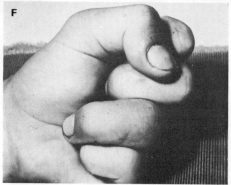

Figure 10–13. *A*, X ray of a fracture of proximal phalanx seen five weeks after injury. The finger had been splinted and follow-up X ray not made until just prior to referral. *B*, X rays of postoperative fixation. *C* and *D*, appearance six months later. *E* and *F*, motion two and a half years later.

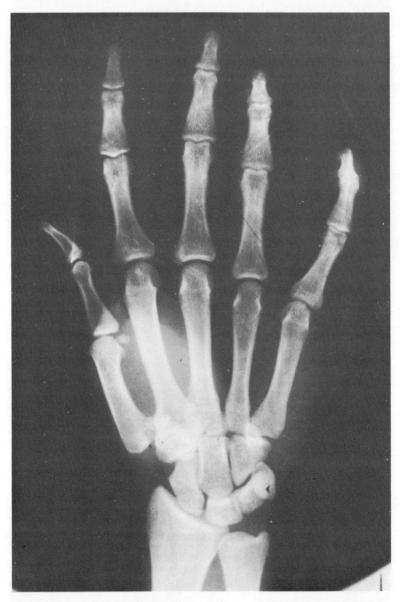

Figure 10–14. X ray showing a fracture at the base of the thumb metacarpal with dislocation of the metacarpal proximal and radialward. The fracture is very unstable, but it is readily reduced by distal traction on the thumb. Accurate reduction and fixation is mandatory for normal thumb function. A Kirschner wire should be drilled through the first metacarpal into the second after reduction.

distal metacarpal may be used. I prefer to use internal fixation to the base of the second metacarpal, with the fracture well reduced by distal traction and by radial pressure over the base of the metacarpal. With the normal relationships at the base of the first metacarpal restored and secured by Kirschner wire, a simple cast immobilizing the thumb for four to five weeks is usually adequate. At the end of this time the cast and Kirschner wire are removed and active movement started.

Figure 10—14 shows a typical Bennett's fracture in a nineteen-year-old man who injured his hand in a fall. The base of the thumb metacarpal is seen to ride proximally and radially. This was treated in the manner just noted. Good reduction was obtained by distal traction, and this was maintained with Kirschner wire fixation to the second metacarpal and with a cast for five weeks. Good function returned following treatment.

METACARPAL FRACTURES

For fractures of the finger metacarpals and the thumb metacarpal away from the carpometacarpal joint, the general principles associated with the phalanges apply. Motion to prevent joint stiffening is mandatory. If the fracture is unstable, cross-pinning with Kirschner wires is best so that the adjacent joints can be kept moving.

Figure 10—15A shows the X ray of a fifty-nine-year-old man who had been struck on the back of the hand by a chair hoist two weeks earlier. The fracture of the index and long finger metacarpals had been immobilized over a roll of gauze in the palm, which is not considered adequate. Three transverse open wounds were present on the back of the hand, which was very swollen. The hand was becoming very stiff. The wounds of the hand were exercised on the following day and secondary closure carried out. With antibiotics, healing occurred. Open reduction of the metacarpal with internal fixation, as shown in figure 10—15B, was then carried out fourteen days later through a fresh incision. Motion of the fingers was instituted at that time. Six months later he had complete flexion of his fingers with only a few degrees limitation of extension. Salvage of movement is credited to the prompt closure of the open wounds and the internal fixation of the metacarpal fractures which allowed finger movement to be carried out. It would have been far safer if this treatment had been carried out at the time of original injury.

Injuries of the joint surface, although quite painful, may be difficult to see in an X ray if the bone fragment is small. Figure 10—16

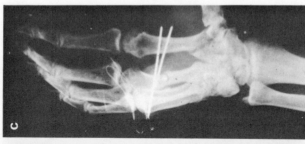
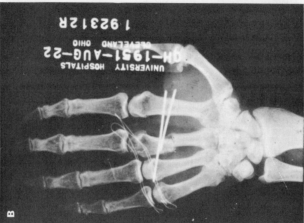
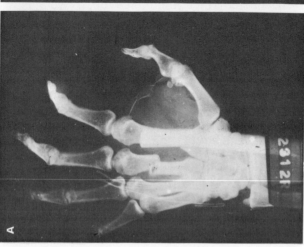

Figure 10–15. *A*, X ray showing the position of metacarpal fractures two weeks after insecure immobilization on a roll of gauze. The hand is very swollen. Open wounds were present on the back of the hand. The wounds were excised and closed the day after the patient was first seen. *B* and *C*, internal fixation was carried out through a fresh incision two weeks later and motion of the fingers emphasized to overcome the joint stiffening, which was becoming severe.

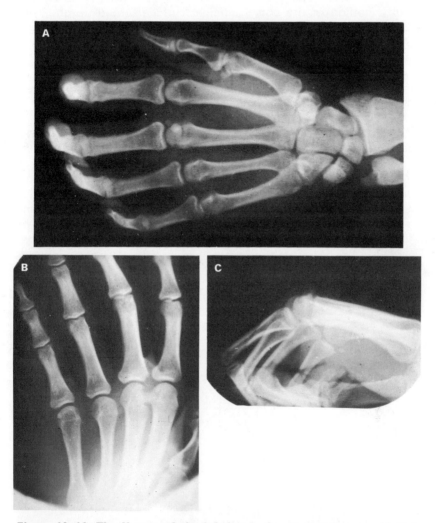

Figure 10–16. The X rays of the left hand of a seventeen-year-old high school football player showing swelling and limited movement of the M-P joint of the long finger two and a half months after being stepped on with a football cleat. Note the dense shadow in *A* at the head of the long finger metacarpal which is shown even better on the oblique and lateral views in *B* and *C*. Oblique and lateral views show the broken articular surface of the long finger metacarpal. Excision of the displaced fragment of articular surface successfully relieved the pain.

shows such a case. The original X ray made two months previously had been falsely interpreted as a sesamoid bone over the distal long finger metacarpal head, a most unlikely diagnosis. Subsequent films (figure 10–16*B* and *C*) showed the true nature of the lesion, with a portion of the dorsal articular surface turned up and lying vertically under the extensor tendon. This was removed surgically, following which the pain subsided and movement improved greatly.

ROTATIONAL DEFORMITY AND OVERLAP OF FINGERS

The teamwork of digits in hand function is manifested in many ways. The thumb works opposite the fingers, increasing their function by pulp-to-pulp apposition. The fingers function side by side in close association, one complementing and augmenting the function of the other. The close proximity of the fingers in flexion makes the plane of this action quite important in preventing interference and overlapping. The eccentric arrangement of the

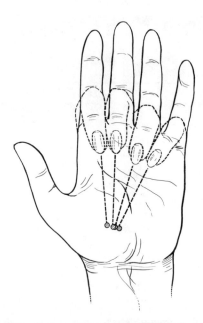

Figure 10–17. The fingers lose most of their lateral mobility and normally converge to comfortable adjacent positions in flexion, as shown by the dotted lines. These planes of flexion are very sensitive to rotational deformity, which may cause the fingers to overlap.

collateral ligaments of the metacarpal heads causes them to tighten in flexion, allowing very little lateral mobility. This makes the accuracy of restoration of the plane of flexion even more important. It should be remembered that as the metacarpal bones diverge from their bases distally, in reverse fashion the fingers converge upon flexion back to the bases of the metacarpals, as shown in figure 10–17. The fingertips can be widely spread when the fingers are extended, allowing independent action, but they are comfortable against one another in the flexed position. This is a beneficial arrangement. In the absence of webbing, money and other objects do not fall through the fingers when the hand is closed, but, in the flexion necessary to provide this, independent lateral movement of the fingers is nearly lost.

Minor degrees of rotation which are enough to cause finger overlap may not be readily visible in an X ray (figure 10–18) and are not visible by inspection when the fingers are extended; yet they are obvious when the fingers are flexed. The plane of the fingernails gives some indication of such deformity, but the most important way to avoid overlap is to place the fingers in the position they should have when the hand is closed. *Since overlap occurs in flexion, it should be recognized and avoided by placing the fingers in flexion.* The splint shown in figure 10–2 provides for this.

Figure 10–18*A* shows the left hand of a thirty-six-year-old man who had fractured the metacarpal of his left right finger four weeks earlier while tussling with his children. The finger had been treated in a cast with the fingers straight. When the cast was removed a week before he was first seen, the ring finger overlapped the small finger, as shown in figure 10–18*B*. It was uncomfortable when he closed his fingers, and he was very unhappy with the result. Note in the X ray, figure 10–18*A*, how little the rotation of the metacarpal head is visible. This X ray was reported as showing excellent alignment. However, with the fingers in flexion, the deformity is readily visible, constituting a much better method of determining adequate reduction. Since the fracture was already firmly healed, a 20° rotatory osteotomy was carried out at the base of the metacarpal where the bone is more cancellous, and internal fixation was utilized, as shown, so that motion could be restored to the fingers a few days after operation.[4] Figure 10–18*C* shows the appearance after rotational osteotomy at the base of the metacarpal, and figure 10–18*D* and *E* show the result two weeks after operation. The Kirschner wires were removed six weeks after operation.

Rotational osteotomy at the base of the metacarpal where healing is usually quite prompt and where internal fixation allows early motion can also be utilized to good advantage for rotational malunion of the phalanx.

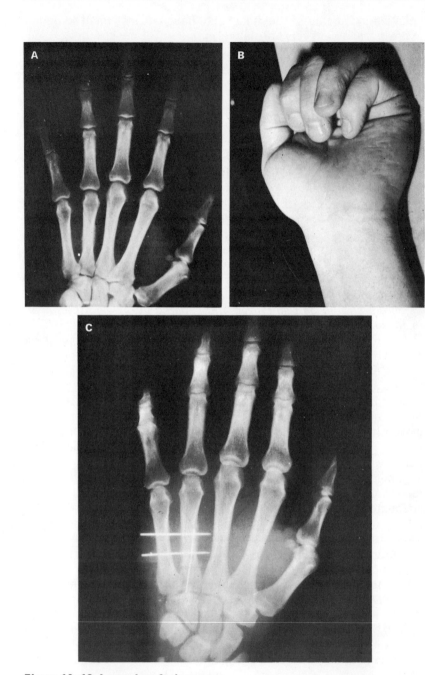

Figure 10–18. Legend on facing page.

Figure 10–19*A* and *B* show the right hand of a fifty-year-old executive who had sustained fractures of the proximal phalanges of the long and ring fingers six months earlier when struck by a golf club. Immobilization had been in the straight position in this patient also. The ring finger had healed with rotational deformity, as shown, so that it crossed under the long finger on flexion. There was joint stiffness and adherence of flexor tendons of the long and ring fingers. Corrective osteotomy of the proximal phalanx would have led to further joint stiffening and tendon adherence. To avoid this, flexor tendolysis was carried out for the two fingers and a 30° rotatory osteotomy performed at the base of the ring metacarpal, with internal fixation, as shown in figure 10–19*C*. Motion was started immediately postoperatively. The Kirschner wires were removed two months after operation. Figure 10–19*D*, *E*, and *F* show his functional result six months later. The finger is still crooked

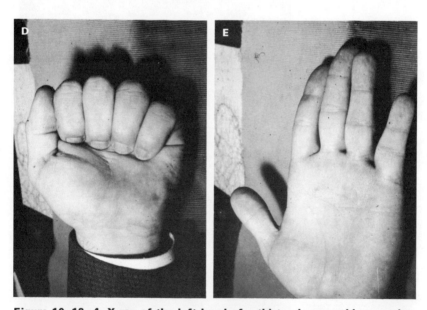

Figure 10–18. *A*, X ray of the left hand of a thirty-six-year-old man taken four weeks after fracture of ring finger metacarpal. Note the apparently good alignment. *B*, on making a fist, the patient has finger overlap. If the fingers had been treated in flexion originally, this deformity would have been obvious and could have been easily corrected by rotation with proper alignment. *C*, X ray showing that the metacarpal rotation had been overcome by osteotomy at its base with internal pin fixation to allow very early movement of the fingers. *D* and *E*, movement present two weeks after operation. (Reproduced, by permission, from Weckesser, Rotational osteotomy of the metacarpal for overlapping fingers. J. Bone Joint Surg. 47-A:751–56, 1965)

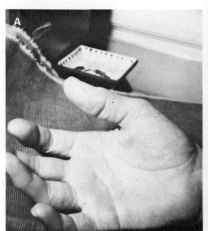
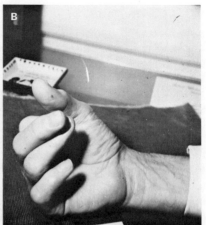
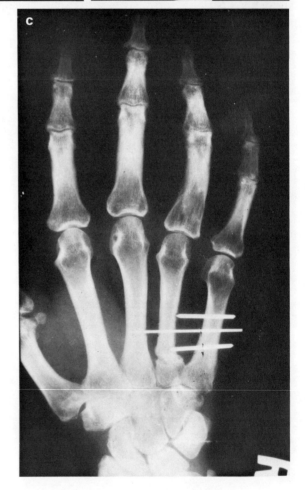

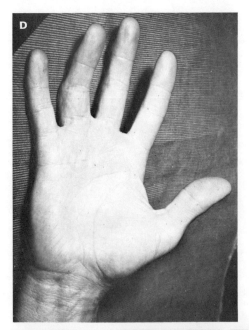

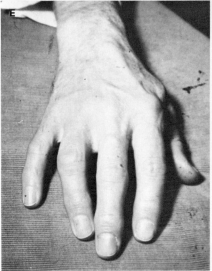

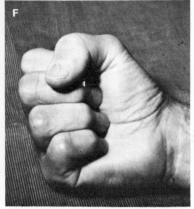

Figure 10–19. *A,* overlapping fingers and limited flexion six months after fracture of proximal phalanges of long and ring fingers. *B,* the rotation is in the proximal phalanx of the ring finger. The flexor tendons are adherent over the former fracture sites. *C,* postoperative X ray following rotational osteotomy of 30°. *D, E,* and *F,* functional result six months later. The patient has painless movement six years later. (Reproduced, by permission, from Weckesser, Rotational osteotomy of the metacarpal for overlapping fingers. J. Bone Joint Surg. 47-A:751–56, 1965)

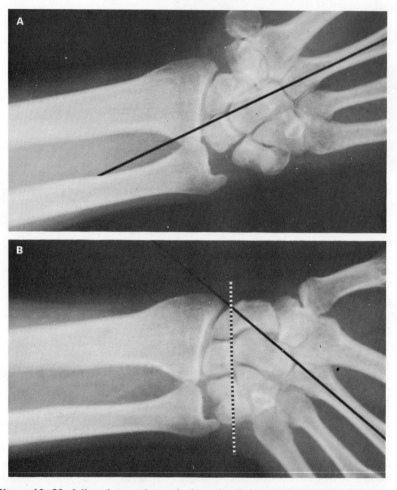

Figure 10–20. A line drawn through the axis of the third metacarpal crosses the carpal lunate bone with the wrist in radial deviation (A) and transects the carpal navicular with the wrist in ulnar deviation (B), showing the cumulative amount of intercarpal movement that occurs.

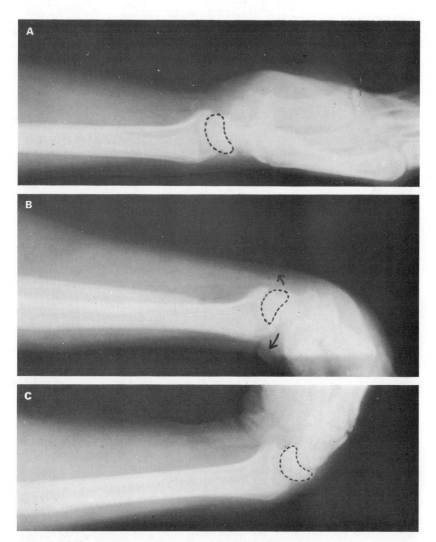

Figure 10–21. When the wrist is forcefully dorsiflexed, the lunate bone may dislocate volarly or the distal row of carpals may dislocate dorsally with a fracture of the navicular (perilunate dislocation).

in extension, but this is a passive movement. When he closes his hand the fingers fit side by side nicely and function with comfort six years later. It is considered that 30° rotation is about the maximum phalangeal rotation that can be corrected by this means.

FRACTURE AND DISLOCATION OF THE WRIST BONES

Movement at the wrist occurs not only at the radiocarpal articulations but between the eight carpal bones themselves. Though the movement between any two carpal bones is not great, the additive effect is significant. As shown in figure 10–20 and as pointed out by Kaplan[2] and by Wagner,[3] a line drawn in the axis of the third metacarpal transects the navicular with the hand in ulnar deviation and falls through the lunate with the hand in radial deviation, because of intercarpal movement. Note also that the intercarpal spaces are visible and essentially equal in width. If the proximal row of carpal bones is considered to be the lunate, the triquetrum, and the pisiform while the distal row is the two multangulars (capitate and hamate), the navicular can be considered the connecting link between the two rows. It is seen that the plane of the midcarpal joint (see figure 10–20) transects the navicular bone. This is the reason that navicular fractures are common and that they are sometimes associated with dislocations at the midcarpal joint, so-called perilunar dislocations. The lunate bone, with its volar portion wider than the dorsal portion, tends to dislocate volarward when the wrist is forcefully dorsiflexed (figure 10–21B). If the lunate maintains its relationship with the radius, the distal row of carpals may dislocate dorsally, once again giving a perilunar dislocation. The mobility of the carpal bones varies, and those persons with more mobility in their proximal row of carpals are probably more prone to have lunate dislocations.

A fencing instructor noted bothersome clicking in his wrist. Multiple views of the wrist showed that this occurred at the navicular lunate articulation because of the laxity at that joint. No treatment was recommended. He probably is more susceptible to lunate dislocation because of this laxity, however.

Figure 10–22A and B show the wrist X rays of a thirty-nine-year-old steel cutter who had sustained severe dorsiflexion of his left wrist when a pressure can which he was holding exploded as the cutter blade transected it. He noted swelling and extreme pain in his wrist immediately after injury, which became progressively worse. The hand and wrist were very swollen and tense when seen twenty-four hours later, at the time this X ray was made. Notice in the anteroposterior view that the intercarpal spaces of the proximal row of carpals are quite altered. On the lateral view, the volar position of the lunate is obvious.

Figure 10–22C shows the wrist with nineteen pounds of traction applied through finger cots over the index and ring fingers. (Note the separation of the M-P joints of these fingers.) With this amount of traction, volar pressure on the displaced lunate has caused it to return to its normal position. A transverse fracture of the triquetrum is also present. The wrist was immobilized in slight flexion by a plaster cast for six weeks. One year later this patient's wrist was asymptomatic.

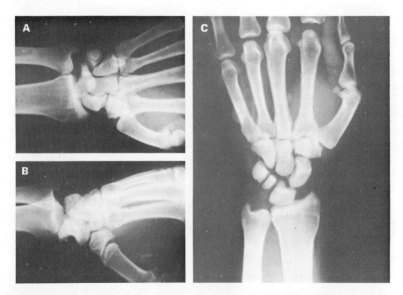

Figure 10–22. X ray of the left wrist twenty-four hours after extreme, forceful dorsiflexion. The patient was having severe pain and swelling. Note the altered intercarpal spaces of the proximal carpal bones in the anteroposterior view (A). The dislocated lunate bone can readily be seen in the lateral view (B). X ray of the left wrist with nineteen pounds traction applied is shown (C). The lunate bone has been reduced by volar pressure. There is also a fracture of the triquetrum.

Figure 10–23A shows a fracture of the left carpal navicular bone that a nineteen-year-old student sustained in a fall on his outstretched hand during athletics six weeks previously. The patient had complained of continued soreness in the radial portion of his left wrist and had tenderness in the anatomical snuffbox. Rarefaction at the fracture site was present. Note that the undisplaced fracture corresponds to the level of the midcarpal joint at the point where stress on the navicular is greatest on forced dorsiflexion of the wrist. It is this same stress which produces movement at the fracture site on wrist motion and that causes nonunion of this bone so frequently if the wrist is not immobilized.

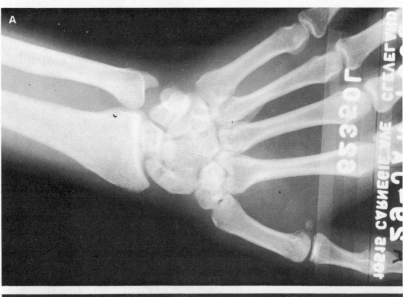

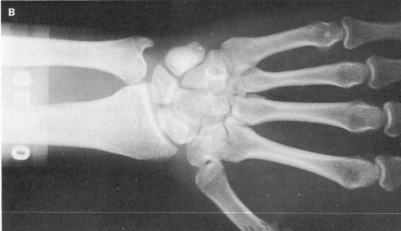

Figure 10–23. *A*, X ray of the right hand showing a fracture of the carpal navicular six weeks after a fall. *B*, healing after four months of immobilization in a plaster cast.

Figure 10–23*B* shows the navicular well healed four months later, after immobilization, including the thumb, in a plaster wrist gauntlet.

An extreme example of fracture dislocation at the midcarpal joint level is shown in figure 10–24*A*. This young man sustained extreme injuries when struck by an automobile. Figure 10–24*B* shows reduction with traction and immobilization in plaster with a transverse Kirschner wire through the metacarpals to give better stability.

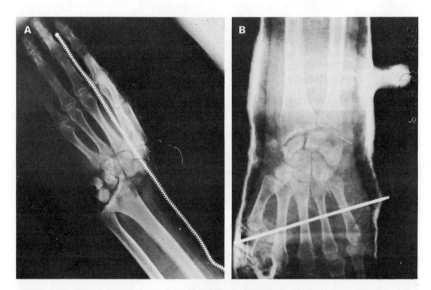

Figure 10–24. *A*, X ray of a compound dislocation of the wrist at the midcarpal joint level. The patient was struck by an automobile. *B*, appearance after reduction by traction and plaster fixation, including a transverse metacarpal pin.

Figure 10–25 shows a fracture of the greater multangular with displacement caused by a cornpicker roller injury. This, as well as the fracture of the ring finger middle phalanx, was reduced by open operation and pinned with Kirschner wires for five weeks. One year later the patient had a painless wrist and hand.

Fractures and dislocations of the carpal bones should be treated at the earliest possible time after injury by reduction and fixation. External fixation by plaster cast is usually sufficient. Traction, as demonstrated in figure 10–22, usually allows ready reduction. Any carpal bone may be fractured. The navicular bone is most frequent since it spans the midcarpal joint and is subject to excessive strain.

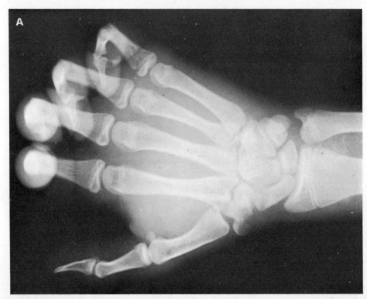

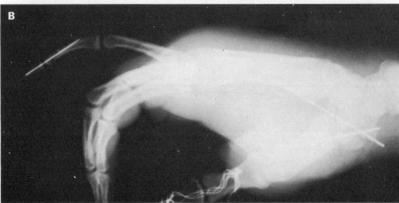

Figure 10–25. Cornpicker injury with fracture of the greater multangular and ring finger proximal phalanx. *A*, A-P view. *B*, lateral view.

This fracture should be immobilized by a cast which stabilizes the wrist and thumb until radiographic union occurs. A navicular fracture is very subject to nonunion if this is not adequately carried out, since the midcarpal joint is prone to produce motion at the site of fracture. Nonunion of the carpal navicular bone gives a painful wrist, and it should be avoided by prolonged immobilization during the primary treatment of the break. Bone grafting is sometimes beneficial in late cases, but it does not always solve the problem by any means—which emphasizes the need for adequate immobilization during the primary treatment of the injury.

Bibliography

1. Aitken, Alexander P.: Fractures of the epiphyses of the upper extremity, in Flynn, J. Edward (ed.): *Hand Surgery*, p. 164 (Baltimore: Williams & Wilkins Co., 1966).
2. Kaplan, Emanuel B.: *Functional and Surgical Anatomy of the Hand*, p. 219 (Philadelphia: J. B. Lippincott Co., 1953).
3. Wagner, Carruth J.: Fracture-dislocations of the wrist, Clin. Orthop. 15:181–96, 1959.
4. Weckesser, Elden C.: Rotational osteotomy of the metacarpal for overlapping fingers, J. Bone Joint Surg. 47-A:751–56, 1965.

CHAPTER 11

Treatment of Infections of the Hand

ABSTRACT

Infections of the hand occur frequently because of the great exposure of the hand to injuries which act as portals of entry for invading organisms. Systemic infection may occur, but, more frequently, the local effects are most troublesome. Function may be crippled, especially by destruction of the gliding mechanism of tendons, joints, and periarticular tissues and by scar formation.

All wounds about the hand should be given special attention because of the hazard of infection here. Cleansing and debridement should be carefully done. If the wound is seen early after injury and is clean, primary closure is indicated. Splinting and prophylactic antibiotics are indicated in wounds entering tendon sheaths and joints particularly. If unusual contamination is present, as in bite and some street wounds, the wound should be left open *after the cleansing process (see chapters 1 and 4). Also, high-velocity gunshot wounds and blast wounds should not be closed, mainly because of the wide area of devitalized tissue which cannot be accurately determined at first treatment.*

Look for foreign bodies in every wound.

Heat, rest, elevation, antibiotics, frequent observation, and early surgery are the framework of the proper treatment of established infection in the hand. Do not wait for fluctuation of pus.

The choice of antibiotic should be made empirically until culture reports are available. The majority of hand infections are caused by gram-positive organisms. A gram stain of the wound should be made to verify this when possible. Erythromycin, lincomycin, sodium methicillin, and sodium oxacillin, at present, are good antibiotics to start with. I prefer erythromycin because of its low incidence of side effects. Chloramphenicol is effective, but it should be used with caution.

Gram-negative organisms are most frequently sensitive to polymyxin B sulfate, colistin, kanamycin sulfate, and chloramphenicol. Sodium ampicillin has a broad spectrum of effectiveness for gram-negative organisms, and so does cephalothin.

With the institution of antibiotics, observation of the infected area should be made every few hours. This requires hospitalization in most instances. If the response is not prompt, incision and drainage along skin lines to prevent the spread of the pus is indicated. The most appropriate antibiotic should be continued until the infection is well under control.

Anaerobic infections are prevented by careful debridement and by leaving wounds open which have been heavily contaminated. Tetanus antitoxin should be administered as well as antibiotics. Certain conditions such as gout, foreign bodies, viral infections, and neoplasia may resemble infection. Neoplasia should be recognized by biopsy.

Pitfalls

1. *Embedded dirt and other foreign bodies*
2. *Deeper wound than anticipated. (The depth cannot be judged by the external appearance.)*
3. *Tendon sheath or joint penetration*
4. *Bite or tooth wounds about M-P joints of fingers*
5. *Lacerations across volar flexion creases of fingers. (The distance to the tendon sheath is very short here.)*
6. *Waiting for fluctuation of pus*
7. *Delaying antibiotics until culture reports are available*
8. *Failing to make observations every few hours*
9. *Failing to admit patient to the hospital*
10. *Development of tetanus or gas gangrene*
11. *Viral infection, which is not benefited by surgery*
12. *Neoplasia, which should be recognized by biopsy*

Cases in Which Outcome Is Apt to Be Less Than Desirable—Early Referral Advisable

1. *Tendon sheath penetration*
2. *Joint penetration*
3. *Bite or tooth wounds*
4. *Tenosynovitis*
5. *Deep infection:*
   midpalmar space
   thenar space
   web space
   collar-button abscess (superficial and deep spaces joined)
6. *Any infection of long standing*
7. *Osteomyelitis*
8. *Anaerobic infection*
9. *Malignancy*

Microorganisms are important in the balance of nature. They break down dead tissue into elements which are reutilized by plant life. Plants, in turn, are utilized as food by animals and humans. Microorganisms are a "friend of man" in this role, but not entirely. They also invade living tissues and at times may be mortal enemies.

Injuries provide portals of entry for invasive organisms, the unchecked growth of which may have dire effects. Immune and reactive cellular responses within the body usually bring invading organisms under control before serious systemic effects occur. Infections of the hand have the additional potential danger of producing serious damage to local structures. This is particularly true for the gliding surfaces of tendons and the mobility of the many small joints in the area. The unique features of the hand which make infections serious may be summarized as follows:

1. The tissues are tightly packed together.
2. There is no room for fluctuation.
3. Pus spreads along tissue planes because there is no room for expansion.
4. Infection injures the gliding mechanism of tendons and alters the mobility of small joints.
5. Systemic spread may occur.

PROPHYLAXIS OF INFECTIONS OF THE HAND

Prevention is the most valuable protection against infections of the hand but often goes unappreciated because, if successful, there is nothing bad with which to compare it. This is always true for preventive measures. The most realistic way is to make comparison with established serious infection.

Prevention involves early wound care, including cleansing, debridement, removal of foreign bodies, and wound irrigation with normal saline (see chapter 1). Lessening the degree of contamination lessens the likelihood of infection, especially if carried out early. Small cuts about the hand should be cleansed with soap and water and treated with a mild antiseptic such as 70% alcohol or, preferably, an antibiotic ointment such as polymyxin B-bacitracin-neomycin (Neosporin) or bacitracin. Loose wound coverage to prevent contamination is desirable. Wounds should be kept clean until healed.

Formerly it was considered that primary closure of wounds was always necessary. This has given way, to some extent, to the concept of delayed emergency under special circumstances (see chapter 1).

CLASSIFICATION OF INFECTIONS

Infection may be classified according to the tissue involved, the etiology, or the organism producing the infection. Each of these considerations is valuable from the standpoint of treatment. The possible types of infection of the hand on the basis of tissue involvement and etiology (figure 11−1) are listed here.

1. Skin and subcutaneous tissue:
      furuncle
      cellulitis
      lymphangitis
      wound infection
      wound with retained foreign body
2. Paronychia
3. Felon (distal closed-space infection)
4. Subcutaneous abscess
5. Web-space infection
6. Tenosynovitis
7. Deep fascial-space infection
8. Joint infection and osteomyelitis
9. Bite wounds
10. Low-velocity gunshot wounds
11. Blast wounds and high-velocity gunshot wounds
12. Anaerobic infection

Stone et al.[4] have found the following distribution of types among 1,251 hand infections admitted to Cook County Hospital from January, 1965, to July, 1968. These cases constituted 19 percent of the hospital admissions to the hand service during that period of time.

TYPE	NUMBER OF PATIENTS
Cellulitis	346
Paronychia	309
Subcutaneous abscess	229
Infected traumatic wound	147
Felon	96
Acute suppurative tenosynovitis	39
Subcuticular abscess	15
Osteomyelitis	14
Postoperative (clean)	7
Miscellaneous	49
TOTAL	1,251

These cases were considered severe enough to be admitted to the hospital. Minor infections were not included. The first five types of infection accounted for 90 percent of the infections.

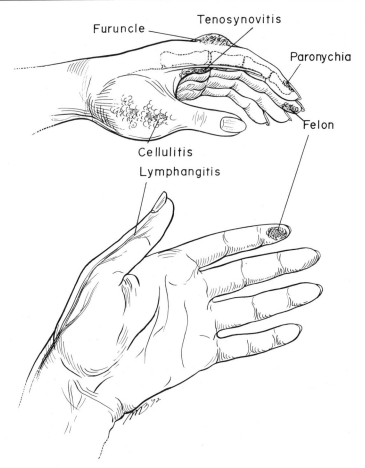

Figure 11–1. Some of the more frequent types of infection about the hand.

TREATMENT OF HAND INFECTIONS

The following procedures are important in treating infections of the hand (see figure 11–2).

1. Heat (to increase blood supply to area)
2. Elevation (to increase venous and lymphatic return, and to diminish swelling)
3. Rest (to lessen spread)
4. Antibiotics
5. Early incision and drainage (do not await fluctuation):
   to diminish pressure
   to prevent further spread
   to remove toxic products

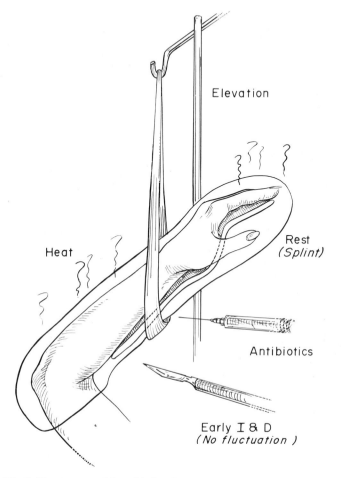

Figure 11–2. Treatment of hand infections.

Heat, rest, and elevation are time-honored, but should be combined with a wise choice of antibiotic before early incision and drainage and before culture reports are available. Because of the tightness of the tissues in the area, fluctuation should not be awaited; it may never occur.

Stone et al.[4] and, more recently, Eaton and Butsch[1] have emphasized the need for antibiotic treatment in severe hand infections before culture reports and sensitivity studies are available. The results of these two studies are valuable and comparable. More than three-fourths of the organisms identified in each study were gram-positive. Mixed cultures of gram-positive and gram-negative organisms were uncommon except in human bite wounds and in infections associated with drug abuse. Gram stain of the wound drainage was helpful in the empirical choice of an antibiotic.

The gram-positive organisms were most frequently sensitive to lincomycin, erythromycin, sodium methicillin, and chloramphenicol. The gram-negative organisms were somewhat less predictable but were found sensitive most often to polymyxin B sulfate, colistin, kanamycin sulfate, and chloramphenicol. I have noted very few side effects with erythromycin and prefer it as the drug of first choice for gram-positive infections. Sodium methicillin or sodium oxacillin, both effective against resistant staphlococci, are the next choice. Cephalothin is another good drug that is effective against both staphylococci and gram-negative organisms in a high percentage of cases.

Whatever drug is chosen empirically, it is safest to check the culture sensitivities as soon as available, unless the clinical response to treatment is unusually good.

In the early treatment of any hand infection, while rest, heat, and an antibiotic are being employed, the patient should be observed frequently to determine when drainage is necessary. It is best to

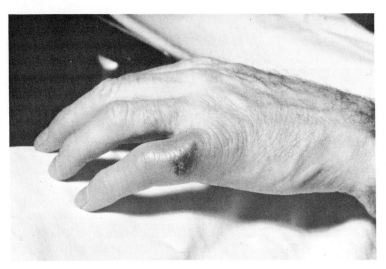

Figure 11–3. Left hand of a forty-eight-year-old physician who noted a furuncle on the dorsum of his small finger ten days earlier which became larger in spite of hot soaks and tetracycline by mouth. Incision and drainage and culture yielded staphylococcus resistant to tetracycline, penicillin, and streptomycin, but sensitive to erythromycin. The antibiotic was changed to erythromycin. After repeated incision and drainage because of progression, the infection came under control. I usually start the patient now on erythromycin, sodium methicillin, or sodium oxacillin.

hospitalize the patient except in mild cases so that hour-by-hour observations are possible. Conditions may change rapidly.

SKIN AND SUBCUTANEOUS TISSUE

The elements of the skin itself may be the seat of infection. This may be severe. If the proper antibiotic is chosen, these infections may respond dramatically, as shown in figure 11–4. Many skin infections are caused by resistant staphylococci (figure 11–3), and it is better to treat them originally with an antibiotic chosen with this in mind.

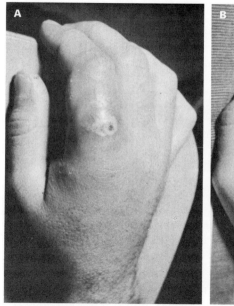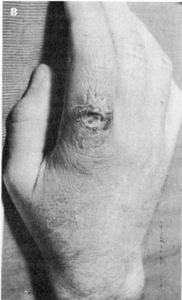

Figure 11–4. Hand of a thirty-three-year-old patient who noted a furuncle (A) which responded to five days of penicillin treatment. This type of response is less frequent than formerly, and it is better to treat originally with erythromycin, sodium methicillin, sodium oxacillin, or lincomycin.

Lymphangitis and cellulitis may be due to a streptococcus infection which usually responds to penicillin G (benzylpenicillin).

All wounds should be carefully cleansed with a mild detergent as soon as possible after injury and irrigated with a large amount of sterile saline solution. Dead tissues should be removed and foreign bodies sought and removed (see figure 11–5). Cleansing the wound

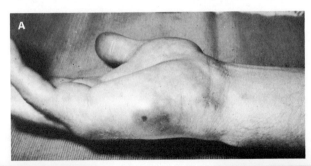

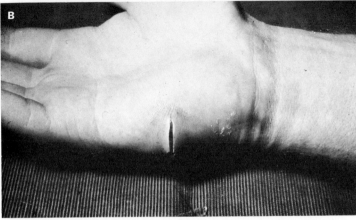

Figure 11–5. *A*, right hand of a twenty-six-year-old patient who evidenced a redness and soreness of the ulnar border. He had put his hand through a storm door five months earlier and the wound had been sutured elsewhere. *B*, incision and drainage yielded pus and fragments of glass, the largest $1\frac{1}{2} \times 2$ cm. Following this, the wound healed promptly. Foreign bodies should be sought in every traumatic wound.

reduces the number of organisms introduced and greatly reduces the chance of infection. When the wound enters a tendon sheath or joint, prophylactic antibiotic is wise (see chapter 1 on primary wound care).

PARONYCHIA

Paronychia, or the growth of organisms—frequently staphylococci —about the margin of the nail, is one of the most common infections of the hand. It may result from any small break in the skin (hangnail) or small puncture wound. The infection usually leads to pus formation at the margin of the nail which can spread laterally or beneath the nail because the eponychium is sealed to the nail. Most of these infections can be aborted if the edge of the eponychium is pushed back with a scalpel blade to break the seal between eponychium and fingernail at the earliest possible time. If pus has formed beneath the nail, the devitalized portion must be removed (see figure 11–6).

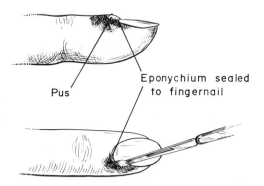

Pus

Eponychium sealed to fingernail

Figure 11–6. Infections under the eponychium, at or under the margin of the nail, are held in by the tight seal of the eponychium to the fingernail. This seal can be broken during the early stages of infection by pushing back the eponychium with a scalpel blade, allowing pus to extrude. If this is done early, the infection will clear. Later, incision must be made as diagrammed by the dotted line in figure 11–12e. If the nail has been elevated by pus, the devitalized portion should be removed.

FELON

Unchecked infection in the tip of any digit may lead to destruction of the distal phalanx (osteomyelitis) (see figure 11–8). To avoid this, early adequate incision of the distal closed space of the digit should be carried out. The patient should be started on an antibiotic empirically, the organism cultured, sensitivity tests made, and the adequacy of the antibiotic checked as soon as test results are available.

Figure 11–7 is a diagram of the fingertip. Incisions should be kept high near the nail. The location of the incision is usually dictated by the location of the infection. The incision should be carried beyond the infected area to give adequate drainage. In severe infections, such as that shown in figure 11–8, a duckbill or fishmouth incision is necessary. By keeping this incision high, the volar flap falls back into place during the healing process, leaving the pad of the digit unscarred. Lesser (earlier) infections do not need this extensive

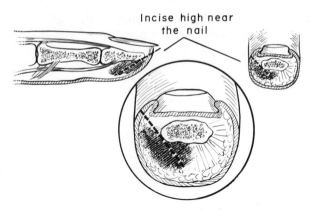

Incise high near
the nail

Figure 11–7. The tip of each digit is a closed pocket in which infection causes pressure and ischemia. If this is to be avoided, liberal incision should be made early. Keep the incision high to leave the pad of the digit unscarred as much as possible.

incision. Usually, adequate drainage can be obtained on one side of the tip only. A small rubber tissue drain introduced into the wound to hold the skin edges apart is important. Frequent observations to check the adequacy of the drainage should be made until the infection is under control.

SUBCUTANEOUS ABSCESS AND WEB-SPACE INFECTION

The subcutaneous and web-space areas are frequent sites of serious infection. Usually, web-space infection is an extension of subcutaneous abscess. The skin acts as a barrier, and pus burrows along the plane of least resistance. One of these routes is along the lumbrical tendon through the lumbrical canal to the dorsum of the finger. This constitutes the so-called web-space infection.

Figure 11–9 is a typical example of a subcutaneous abscess which extended laterally and dorsally. Pus was under pressure when released. Fluctuation of the pus did not occur because of the tight arrangement of the structures of the palm. Counterincisions were made over the proximal phalanges of the ring and small fingers, in addition to the fourth web space, to insure proper drainage. The organism was *Staphylococcus aureus*, sensitive to nearly all antibiotics, but partially resistant to sodium ampicillin. The infection subsided promptly after drainage. Earlier drainage would have diminished the spread and created less risk. A wisely chosen antibiotic, used very early, might have aborted the infection.

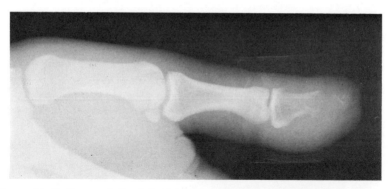

Figure 11–8. X ray of the left thumb of a twenty-nine-year-old man who developed soreness and swelling of the tip three weeks earlier. The thumb had been opened on two occasions, but it had not drained adequately nor had it been determined or recognized that the organism was a staphylococcus resistant to penicillin. On the day this X ray was made, the thumb was still swollen and red, with pus exuding from two small incisions through the skin. Culture of the pus was made. The patient was given erythromycin and admitted to the hospital, and the thumb opened widely around the tip close to the nail to expose the necrotic distal phalanx, which was then curetted away. The organism was found sensitive to erythromycin, which was continued. The wound was packed open and allowed to heal from its base. The final scar close to the thumbnail, and the pulp of the digit has good sensation. This case of osteomyelitis could have been prevented by a wiser choice of antibiotic and wider surgical incision earlier.

TENOSYNOVITIS

Infection in the sheaths about flexor tendons, tenosynovitis, is a serious complication of any cut of the volar surface of the digit, particularly a cut which crosses the flexion crease. The distance between skin and tendon sheath at the flexion crease is only a few millimeters. Any wound entering a tendon sheath should be cleansed and irrigated with large amounts of saline solution. I place a patient with this type of wound on prophylactic antibiotic, such as erythromycin (250 mgm q.i.d.), and observe the patient closely, preferably by admission to the hospital. Pain is a danger-sign.

If infection in this location is not recognized and treated early, the gliding mechanism of the tendon will be destroyed.

The classical symptoms of the tendon sheath infection of the finger are that:

1. The finger is held in flexion.
2. It is tender along the course of the tendon sheath.
3. Severe pain occurs when it is extended.

When this diagnosis is suspected to be so, the patient should be hospitalized, appropriate antibiotic begun, and early incision and

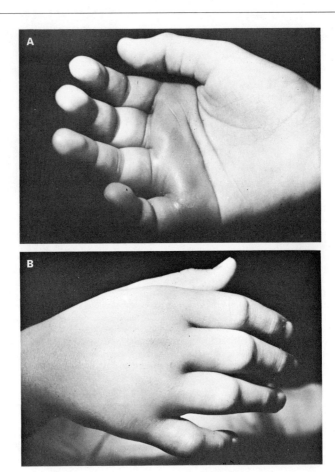

Figure 11–9. Right hand of a twelve-year-old boy who had developed a blister at the base of his ring finger fourteen days earlier while chopping down a tree. The edge of the blistered skin pulled loose five days prior to these photos, following which progressive swelling and redness developed in spite of hot soaks and sodium ampicillin by mouth. The photos show the swelling of the distal palm, fingers, and dorsum of the hand.

drainage carried out unless response to the antibiotic is prompt. Hematogenous tenosynovitis may also occur from gonococcus infection in the genital tract. This type of infection will frequently respond to systemic antibiotic treatment during an eight-hour trial under close observation in the hospital. If response does not occur in this time, incision and drainage should be carried out.

Figure 11–10 shows tenosynovitis secondary to a neglected laceration across the distal flexion crease of the finger. This should have been observed closely and recognized earlier. Wounds entering tendon sheaths are treacherous.

DEEP FASCIAL-SPACE INFECTION

Deep fascial-space infections are not very common. They are most apt to occur after deep puncture wounds which carry organisms deep into the center of the hand around the interosseous muscles (mid-palmar space) or about the adductor muscle of the thumb (thenar space) or deep into the hypothenar muscles. Symptoms of such infection are diffuse swelling and deep tenderness in the palm and back of the hand. Adequate early incision along flexion creases is safest together with appropriate antibiotic therapy (see figure 11 –11).

JOINT INFECTION AND OSTEOMYELITIS

Synovial fluid offers a good culture medium for most organisms. This location of contamination must be considered with all penetrating wounds near joints to prevent the development of pyarthrosis. It is highly important that joint penetration be recognized at the time of occurrence so that the joint can be opened and irrigated freely with sterile saline and placed at rest and so that prophylactic antibiotics can be given. Unchecked pyogenic bacterial growth will destroy the joint cartilage and produce osteomyelitis of the underlying bone. The signs of established joint infection, less specific than for many other types of infection, are:
1. Diffuse swelling and redness about the joint
2. Pain on joint motion
These signs may also occur from surrounding cellulitis. In case of doubt, it is best to explore surgically in a bloodless field to see whether the joint capsule and synovium are distended. Care should be taken not to introduce infection if it is not already there.

Osteomyelitis also gives diffuse and persistent signs of infection which can be identified by X ray after it is established. Wide incision and drainage with appropriate antibiotic treatment should be carried out.

BITE WOUNDS

All bite wounds have a serious potential for infection. Human bite wounds should be cleansed and debrided and left open until the

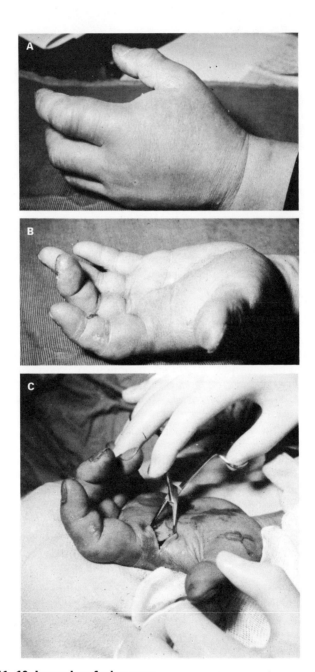

Figure 11-10. Legend on facing page.

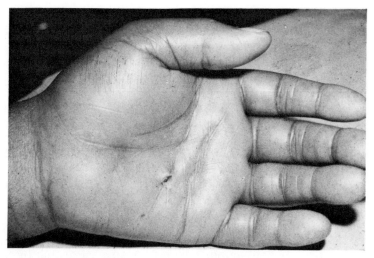

Figure 11–11. Left hand of a seventy-year-old man who presented with tenseness and swelling of the palm which had been punctured with a piece of wood while carving three days earlier. Incision and drainage parallel with the midpalmar crease yielded pus and a wood fragment measuring $\frac{1}{2} \times 4$ cm. Recovery was prompt following wide drainage.

hazard of infection has passed, usually for several days. Prophylactic antibiotic should be given and the patient hospitalized or seen daily for evaluation if the wound is near any important structure. Wounds about the knuckles should be suspected of being human bite wounds from tooth penetration among people who have been fighting. Many of these wounds penetrate the joint, and when the fingers are straightened this track is sealed, increasing the hazard of infection in the joint.

Figure 11–10. A and B, the right hand of a sixty-five-year-old man who punctured the volar aspect of his index finger over the distal flexion crease with a chicken bone while at work making chop suey at a restaurant four days earlier. He continued to work. The finger became progressively swollen and sore. Note that the finger was tensely swollen and held in flexion. There was tenderness along the course of the flexor tendon sheath, and passive extension was very painful, the classical signs of tenosynovitis. C, incision was made in the palm at the base of the finger, and pus was released. When saline was irrigated into this incision, it extruded through the original distal wound at the distal flexion crease. A small polyethylene catheter was inserted into the tendon sheath through which 0.25% neomycin solution was irrigated every three hours. The patient was given sodium oxacillin systemically. The organism was a staphylococcus sensitive to most antibiotics. Response was prompt, and the wound healed with moderate restriction of flexion to two centimeters of the base of the digit eight weeks later.

For established infection, the patient should be hospitalized and heavy doses of an antibiotic effective against resistant staphylococci should be given until culture sensitivities are obtained.

Animal bites can also be serious if neglected and should be treated in a manner similar to human bite wounds. Cats and dogs frequently harbor *Pasteurella multocida*, a gram-negative rod in their mouths which produces cellulitis and which may localize about a tendon, joint, or in a closed fascial space. Fortunately, this organism is sensitive to many antibiotics. Cat bite infection caused by *Pasteurella multocida* is to be distinguished from cat-scratch fever which is caused by a virus. Hawkens[3] found *Pasteurella multocida* in the mouths of 52 percent of 100 healthy cats and dogs (see chapter 1).

LOW-VELOCITY GUNSHOT WOUNDS

Low-velocity bullet wounds create their greatest danger by transecting deep structures and carrying surface dirt and clothing into the wound, which produce infection.

It is best to open any wound which penetrates a joint or tendon sheath, debride it, remove foreign bodies, irrigate it freely, and treat it with prophylactic antibiotics. Secondary closure can be carried out in several days if the wound is large; if the wound is small, it will heal spontaneously.

The through-and-through bullet track which does not transect important structures (tendons, nerves, blood vessels) should be debrided from each end, irrigated freely, treated with antibiotic, splinted, and allowed to heal (see also chapter 1).

HIGH-VELOCITY GUNSHOT WOUNDS AND BLAST WOUNDS

The destruction from high-velocity gunshot wounds and blast wounds is so severe that debridement should be wide and the wound treated open. Subsequent debridement may be necessary. Closure or coverage by skin graft or pedicle should be carried out after the wound appears healthy (see chapter 1).

INCISIONS FOR INFECTION

Incisions parallel to skin lines and folds are most desirable when and if they give adequate exposure of the infected area (see figure 11–12). In general, drainage incisions should be liberal to drain the

a) Parallel creases in palm
b) Cross a cleft vertically
c) Midlateral incision of digit
d) Felon incision kept high
e) Paronychia parallel with
      margin of nail

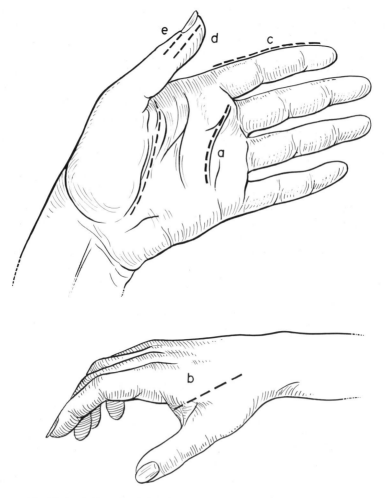

Figure 11–12. Incisions for infections.

margins of the infected area. This is particularly true when the organism is resistant to the antibiotic in use. The midlateral incision gives wide exposure in the finger when this is necessary. Proximal and distal irrigation for tenosynovitis through small incisions into the tendon sheath at either end has been found helpful. Small polyethylene catheters inserted at either end can be used to introduce antibiotic solution for irrigation at frequent intervals.

TETANUS AND GAS GANGRENE

The hazard of life-threatening anaerobic infections, such as tetanus and gas gangrene, in penetrating wounds of the upper extremity is ever present. Prophylaxis demands great care. Debridement and thorough cleansing of all penetrating wounds is of primary importance. Heavily contaminated wounds should be left open. This should be supplemented by large doses of antibiotic in high-risk cases. Tetanus toxoid should be administered regularly to all patients. If the patient has not been previously immunized with tetanus toxoid, antitoxin—human or animal—should be given.

The treatment of established tetanus or gas gangrene infection demands the highest cooperation of surgeon, anesthesiologist, and internist in a medical center. These grave cases should be transferred as soon as possible to that type of care.

An outline of treatment of persons in various stages of immunity for the prophylaxis of tetanus according to Furste[2] is as follows:

    1. To previously immunized patients
        a. Those who have been immunized or received boosters within the last ten years:
            Besides wound debridement, give 0.5 ml of tetanus toxoid. This is enough, even in serious injuries with obvious risk of tetanus.
        b. Those who have been immunized more than ten years previously:
            In most of these cases, wound debridement and 0.5 ml tetanus toxoid are sufficient.
            In cases where a serious risk of tetanus is suspected, give 250 units of tetanus-immune globulin (human) in addition to 0.5 ml tetanus toxoid.
    2. To unimmunized or only partly immunized patients
        a. Wounds that can be completely cleaned or excised, where the risk of tetanus is considered small:
            Give 0.5 ml tetanus toxoid. This has no effect for the actual injury if the patient has not received any

toxoid earlier. Arrange for the complete immunization of the patient, if this is not his third injection.

b. Wounds where complete wound debridement is not
possible and where the risk of tetanus is considered
to be great:

Give 0.5 ml tetanus toxoid and arrange for the continued immunization program of the patient.
Give 250 units of tetanus-immune globulin
(human). Consider the use of antibiotics. Penicillin and tetracycline can prevent simultaneous
infection with other microorganisms that favor
tetanus spores by creating anaerobic conditions.

CONDITIONS WHICH MAY BE CONFUSED WITH BACTERIAL INFECTION

Gout

Gout is a painful condition that produces redness, swelling, and
tenderness equal to bacterial infection, caused apparently by the
deposition of urate crystals in joint cartilage or snyovium, under
certain poorly understood conditions. The differential diagnosis is
made on the basis of unusual suddenness of onset, absence of a
wound, elevation of the serum uric acid level above 7 mgm per 100
ml, and the usual response to 0.5 mgm colchicine given every two
hours until relief or until diarrhea develops.

Figure 11–13 shows the forearm and hand of a fifty-three-year-
old woman with excruciating pain in the right hand, wrist, and dorsal
forearm. There was extreme swelling which had started two days
earlier. The fingers were held in partial flexion. There was diminished
pinprick sensation of the thumb, index and long fingers. The blood
uric acid level was 8 mgm per 100 ml. A diagnosis of acute snyovitis
with carpal tunnel syndrome was made and immediate surgery carried
out because of the severity of the symptoms and the danger of permanent median nerve damage. The transverse carpal ligament was
divided. There was milky fluid in the tendon sheaths. No growth of
bacteria was present. This severe attack might have been aborted
with colchicine, if it had been given earlier. The drug was not effective during the forty-eight hours preceding surgery. Following
surgery, the patient's pain subsided promptly. Four months later sensation was normal in her hand, her fingers flexed normally, except
the index finger which closed to $1\frac{1}{2}$ cm of the base of the digit. This
was synovitis caused by urate deposition. Acute single joint arthritis

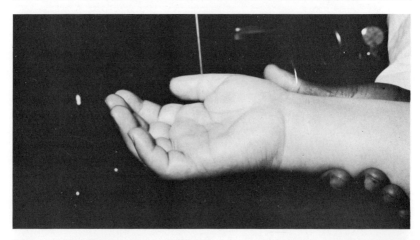

Figure 11–13. **Right hand of a fifty-three-year-old woman who complained of excruciating pain and swelling in the right wrist and hand of five days duration. Blood uric acid was 8 mgm per 100 ml. There was numbness of the thumb, index, and long fingers. Symptoms increased during forty-eight hours of colchicine therapy. At surgery, the transverse carpal ligament was divided. There was milky fluid and inflammation about the flexor tendons and median nerve. There was no evidence of growth of organisms. This case was diagnosed as gouty tenosynovitis with acute carpal tunnel syndrome.**

with redness and swelling, resembling infection, may also occur in the hand.

Foreign Body

Although bacterial infection and a foreign body may coexist, the latter usually produces tenderness and inflammation when it exists alone. Soreness in any wound after healing should raise the suspicion of a retained foreign body (see figure 11–5).

Since foreign bodies produce inflammatory reaction, it is considered wisest to make special effort to remove them, unless they are very small. This is especially true in the hand where the reactions set up by foreign bodies may interfere with normal gliding mechanisms. Every traumatic wound should be carefully inspected for a hidden foreign body, and foreign bodies such as shell fragments and bullets should be removed.

Viral Infection

Viral infection should be recognized because it usually does not benefit from surgical incision and drainage as does bacterial infection. Vesicle formation is usually present in the early stages and should serve to alert the surgeon. Herpes simplex occurs on the digits. I recently took care of a colleague with vaccinia of the end of the index finger, proved by viral culture (see figure 11–14). These conditions are usually best treated by allowing them to run their natural course. The products of suppuration need not be drained as in bacterial infection.

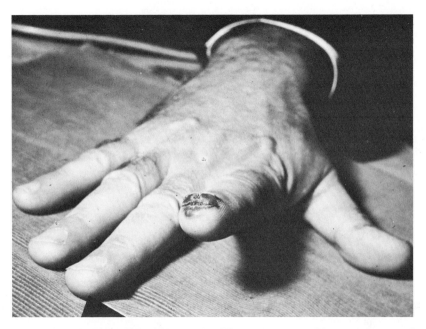

Figure 11–14. Right index finger of a fifty-seven-year-old man who noted redness, swelling, and pain ten days earlier which was associated with swelling of the distal closed space. This progressed rather rapidly, and an incision was made which did not yield pus. Vesicles were present on the skin. These had become largely crusted at the time of this photo, except at the very tip. Vaccinia virus was grown from the wound fluid. The process gradually subsided over the next week.

Neoplasia

Neoplasia, although not frequent, may be present and should be considered in any condition which does not heal.

Figure 11–15 shows an inflamed area of the nail bed of the long finger which had been present one year. Biopsy showed squamous cell carcinoma, and finger amputation was carried out.

Figure 11–16*A* shows the right hand of a sixty-three-year-old dentist who had had inflammation of his long finger for three years.

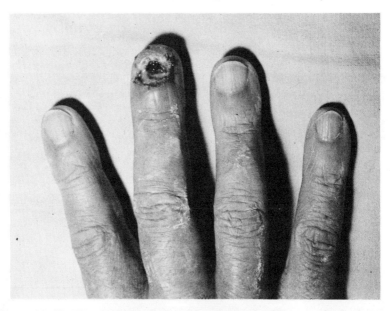

Figure 11–15. The right hand of a fifty-five-year-old man who had noted redness and soreness of the nail bed of the long finger for one year. The nail had been removed, but the inflammed area remained. Biopsy showed squamous cell carcinoma at the time this photo was made. Amputation of the finger was carried out through the proximal phalanx, and the patient was well six years later.

He had been using this finger to hold x-ray films during exposure for dental X rays. Biopsy showed squamous cell carcinoma. The treatment and follow-up are depicted in figure 11–16*B*, *C*, and *D*. He continued to practice dentistry and is well without recurrence thirteen years later.

Figure 11–16. *A*, the right hand of a sixty-three-year-old dentist, who had had inflammation of the long finger for three years. He had held X-ray films with this finger for years during dental X ray exposure. Biopsy showed squamous cell carcinoma. *B*, treatment consisted of amputation of the long finger ray. *C* and *D* are follow-up photographs. He is fine thirteen years later.

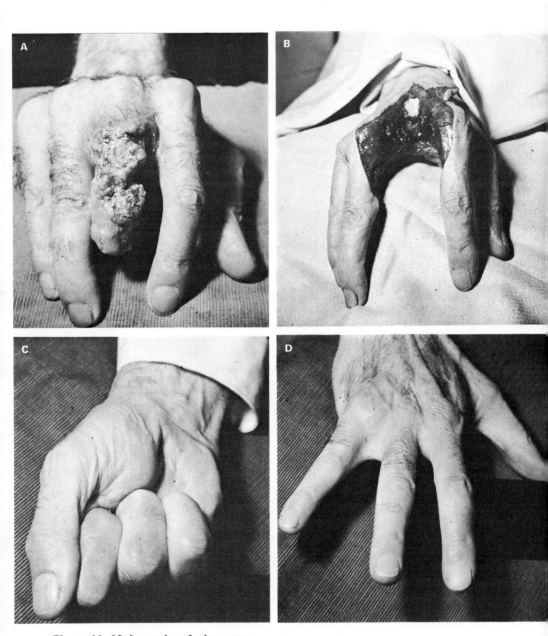

Figure 11–16. Legend on facing page.

Bibliography

1. Eaton, Richard G., and Butsch, David P.: Antibiotic guidelines for hand infections, Surg. Gynecol. Obstet. 130:119–22, 1970.
2. Furste, Wesley: Tetanus: By 1980, a disease of only historical significance in the United States of America, J. Trauma 10: 831–38, 1970.
3. Hawkins, Leland G.: Local *Pasteurella multocida* infections, J. Bone Joint Surg. 51-A:363–66, 1969.
4. Stone, Nelson H.; Hursch, Hester; Humphrey, Charles R.; and Boswick, John A., Jr.: Empirical selection of antibiotics for hand infections, J. Bone Joint Surg. 51-A:899–903, 1969.

CHAPTER 12

Example Cases of Hand Injury

The following cases demonstrate certain problems in the treatment of injuries of the hand. Some are common. Some are unusual. The history of each case, as well as a photograph showing the extent of injury, is given.

Test your skill in diagnosis and treatment.

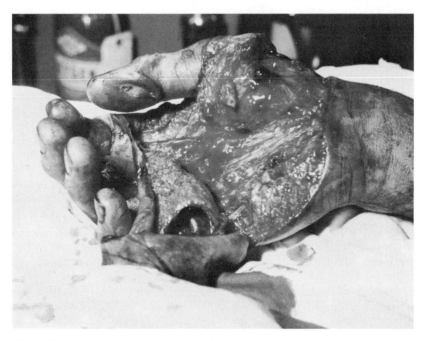

Figure 12–1. See Case 1.

CASE 1—AVULSION INJURY

A nineteen-year-old workman caught his right hand in a printing press. The palmar skin was avulsed distally with attachment still present at the base of the fingers (Figure 12–1). This is an unusual avulsion since this type of injury usually occurs on the dorsum of the hand rather than on the firmly attached palmar skin, which was avulsed in this case.

How should this distally based skin flap be treated?

DISCUSSION OF CASE 1.

Skin flaps with their bases attached distally are noted for their poor vascular supply. Even though circulation may seem adequate shortly after injury, there is a great tendency for late thrombosis of vessels to occur, leading to gangrene. However, it is desirable to preserve as much palmar skin as possible.

At operation, immediately following the photos shown in figure 12–1, the hand was cleansed and the wound irrigated with copious amounts of normal saline solution. The flap was cut back to fresh bleeding and this portion preserved over the distal palm. The proximal portion of the palm was covered with a dermatome skin graft 0.018 inch thick. The preserved skin flap over the distal palm was kept under observation. After several days the central and proximal portions of the flap lost viability. One week after the first operation, the nonviable portion of the flap was excised and a second dermatome graft applied to the center of the palm. The condition of the hand eighteen months after treatment is shown in figure 12–2.

Pedicle replacement of skin and subcutaneous fat would have been an alternate method. This would have involved attachment of the hand to another part of the body for several weeks. It would have been cumbersome, and it is questionable whether the result in this case would have been significantly better. Management of the additional necrosis of the palmar flap would have been difficult had a pedicle been employed.

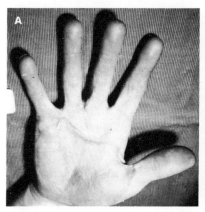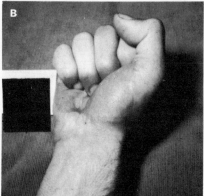

Figure 12–2. Condition of the hand of the patient in figure 12–1 eighteen months after treatment. The area requiring secondary grafting in the center of the palm is visible. The patient carries out his previous type of work. Loss of the normal palmar skin texture (dermal ridges) interferes with some functions; the patient complains that objects slip from his grasp more readily now than before the injury. This is not a serious complaint, however, and he has good use of his hand.

CASE 2—DEEP LACERATION OF FOREARM

A nineteen-year-old student's right hand accidentally went through a glass storm door three weeks before this photo was made. She had extensive lacerations on the volar surface of the midportion of the right forearm with laceration of flexor muscles and embedded fragments of glass. The flexor muscles and the wounds had been repaired on the night of injury. On removal of the splint several days before figure 12—3 was made, it was noted that she could not extend her wrist. She was referred for treatment because of this condition. There is numbness and anesthesia of the dorsum of the thumb and radial border of the distal portion of the index metacarpal.

What is still wrong here?

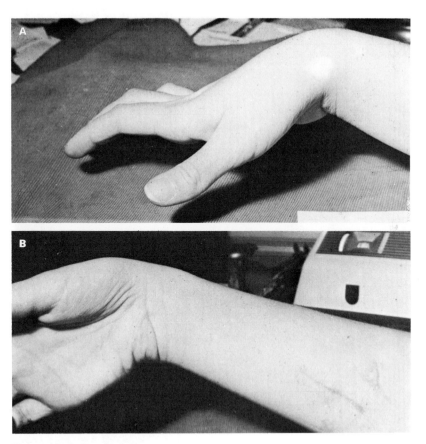

Figure 12—3. See Case 2.

DISCUSSION OF CASE 2.

Examination showed there was no action of the extensor carpi radialis tendon-muscle units. The extensor carpi ulnaris muscle as well as the extensor communis of the fingers and the extensors of the thumb were functioning. The limited sensation in the sensory distribution of the radial nerve indicated injury here.

There are two possibilities that might cause inability to extend the wrist in such a case:

1. Laceration of the motor branch of the radial nerve to the extensor carpi radialis tendons along with laceration of sensory fibers.
2. Laceration of the extensor carpi radialis tendons themselves.

Surgical exploration several days later revealed that the glass spicules from the door had penetrated the interosseous membrane of the forearm and directly divided the radial extensor tendons of the wrist as well as the sensory branches of the radial nerve. The two tendons and the nerve were repaired, and the patient made a good recovery.

CASE 3—LOSS OF FLEXION

A twenty-two-year-old machinist's left hand was caught between a conveyor belt and a punch press five months before figure 12—4 was made. The ring finger, severely mangled, was amputated through the proximal phalanx at a hospital shortly after injury. The wounds healed without infection, but active flexion of the small finger did not return except to the distal joint when the finger was held straight. The long finger did not snug into the palm when the patient attempted to make a fist. Passively, the finger could be pushed into the palm. The joints were not stiff.

What has happened that has caused the loss of normal flexion of his long and small fingers?

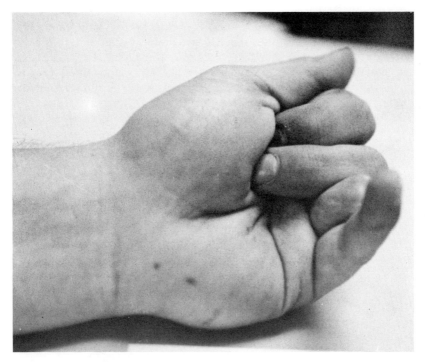

Figure 12—4. See Case 3.

DISCUSSION OF CASE 3.

Possible causes that might result in the loss of normal flexion of the long and small fingers are:

1. Avulsion of the profundus flexor of the small finger.
2. Tear of muscle bellies of the profundus flexors to the long and small fingers.
3. Adhesions of the profundus flexor in the stump of the ring finger, with checkrein effect on excursion of the profundus tendons of the adjacent fingers.

The profundus muscle is usually a single muscle belly with the four profundus tendons coming from it. If one of these tendons is adherent in a finger, excursion in the adjacent fingers is limited by this checkrein effect. If the profundus were avulsed from its insertion in the small finger, there would be no active flexion of the distal joint even with the finger straight. Partial tears of the muscle bellies are possible, but rare.

At surgery, the flexor profundus tendon of the amputated ring finger was found adherent to the proximal phalanx of this digit. It was freed and allowed to retract into the palm. Postoperatively the patient had complete flexion of the long and small fingers. It is important to remember that when a finger is amputated, the flexor profundus tendon should be allowed to retract.

CASE 4—EXTENSION INSTEAD OF FLEXION

On making a fist, this fifty-year-old man's right long finger went into forceful extension instead of flexion (figure 12–5). A tendon graft operation had been done elsewhere four months earlier, three months after an industrial injury in which the flexor tendons of the finger had been lacerated. He also had impaired sensation of the thumb and index finger, and the thenar eminence was flat at the time of the examination. These last two findings had their onset following the tendon graft operation. Flexion of the long finger had never occurred. He stated that the tendency of the finger to straighten had become more pronounced with time.

What would make the finger extend when the others were being flexed, and, why does he unfortunately have sensory impairment as well as a flat thenar eminence?

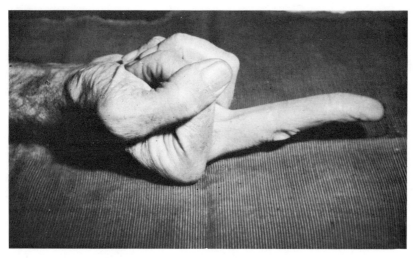

Figure 12–5. See Case 4.

DISCUSSION OF CASE 4.

At operation the median nerve was found grafted into the flexor profundus tendon from palm to fingertip. With the stretching of this structure the lumbrical muscle origin on the profundus tendon had pulled proximal, transmitting unusual force to the extensor hood and straightening the interphalangeal joints of the finger.

Flexor tendon graft utilizing the sublimis tendon was carried out. (*The patient had no palmaris longus tendon*). An opponens transfer operation and nerve graft operation is planned.

CASE 5—LOSS OF FLEXION

A fifty-five-year-old man sustained a cut on the volar aspect of the right small finger, figure 12—6, caused by the sharp edge of a metal box while at work. He had no active flexion of the interphalangeal joints but good flexion of the M-P joint of this digit. Sensation was normal.

What is the reason for his disability, and why is he able still to flex his M-P joint?

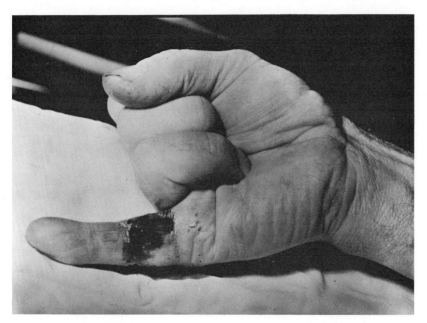

Figure 12—6. See Case 5.

DISCUSSION OF CASE 5.

The disability here is a result of laceration of the flexor profundus and sublimis of the right small finger in Zone II (No Man's Land). Because lumbrical and interossei muscles are intact, he is still able to flex his M-P joint.

Primary treatment involved cleansing, irrigation, and soft tissue closure to obtain healing. Three weeks later a tendon graft utilizing the sublimis tendon to span the area of No Man's Land from palm to fingertip was carried out. Primary repair in this zone often fails, and is best not attempted except by the expert, and then only in ideal cases. For further discussion see chapter 8.

CASE 6—JOINT EXPOSURE

A twenty-four-year-old man caught his right hand while guiding a basket of hot steel ingots. The intense heat burned his right long finger through his asbestos glove while his hand was caught for about one minute and until it could be pried free. This injury occurred eighteen days before figure 12–7 was made. Treatment elsewhere had been expectant. The destruction is into the middle finger joint.

How can the open joint of this finger be saved?

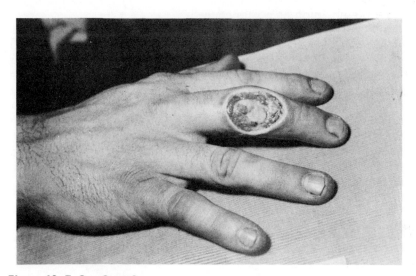

Figure 12–7. See Case 6.

DISCUSSION OF CASE 6.

The wound was debrided and crystallized trypsin powder applied intermittently for twenty-four hours. By these methods, a large number of small bits of devitalized tissue were removed. Four days after admission, a primary abdominal pedicle flap was applied. This was detached three weeks later when it had healed well onto the long finger.

There was slight loss at one edge of the pedicle, but adequate tissue was transferred to cover the defect satisfactorily. Motion was started early to prevent further joint stiffness.

Figure 12–8 shows the appearance of the finger and the range of motion nine months postoperatively.

This patient should have received definitive treatment earlier. The necrosis over the finger joint had been severe and had extended into the joint. The chances of infection here were very great, but there was no alternative but to attempt to cover the open area with a primary skin flap. I chose the abdomen, rather than another area, because the hazard of infection was so great. A cross-finger pedicle flap would have been an alternate method here but would have been fraught with greater danger to the donor digit. Fortunately, the pedicle healed and the joint was preserved. This was a close call and could have been avoided by earlier definitive pedicle treatment.

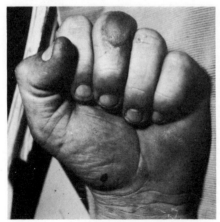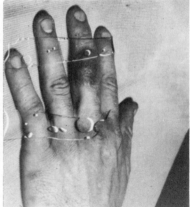

Figure 12–8. Appearance and range of motion of the patient in figure 12–7 nine months postoperatively.

CASE 7—FINGERTIP INJURY

A fifty-three-year-old woman caught her right small finger in an automobile door shortly before figure 12−9 was made. The small finger is amputated through the middle of the fingernail, as shown.

What should be done?

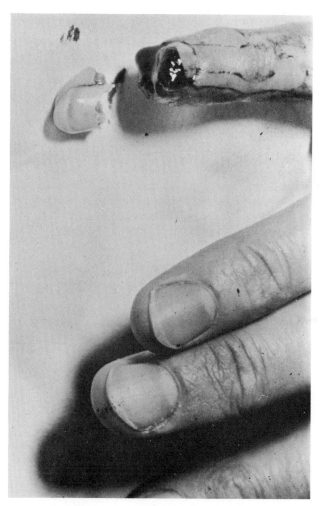

Figure 12−9. See Case 7.

DISCUSSION OF CASE 7.

The subcutaneous tissues were removed from the skin of the amputated tip and the tip resutured over the end of the finger.

Resuture of the tip is usually not successful unless the subcutaneous tissues are removed. If this is done, the skin of the tip can be reapplied as a full-thickness graft—if it is healthy. The ultimate success of free grafting, either of the original tissues or of a fresh free graft, depends upon the amount of soft tissue remaining at the tip of the finger. If there is enough soft tissue left to cover the end of the bone, it is a satisfactory and simple method of solving the problem.

For more complete consideration of this problem, see chapter 7.

CASE 8—CRUSH INJURY OF THUMB

A man caught his right thumb in a punch press shortly before figure 12–10 was made. The thumb was severely crushed, as shown. The distal phalanx and part of the proximal phalanx were severely comminuted.

What is the proper treatment?

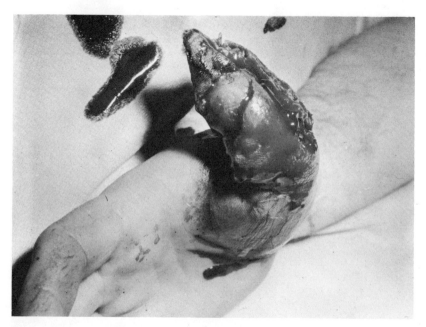

Figure 12–10. See Case 8.

DISCUSSION OF CASE 8.

All viable tissue was preserved. Amputation was necessary through the distal portion of the proximal phalanx. Local flaps were utilized for closure, as shown in figure 12–11. The wounds healed slowly, but a functional short thumb was obtained which had sensation.

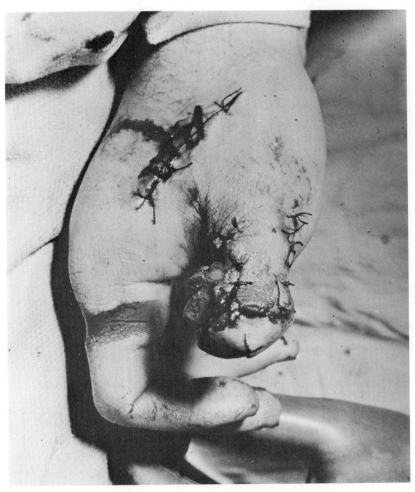

Figure 12–11. A shortened thumb was preserved with adjacent sensitive skin flaps.

CASE 9—FINGER FRACTURE

X ray (figure 12–12) of a fifty-three-year-old man who caught his left long and ring fingers between a belt and a pulley four days previously, while at work. The long finger fracture is still unreduced in spite of previous attempts at reduction made elsewhere.

What should be done?

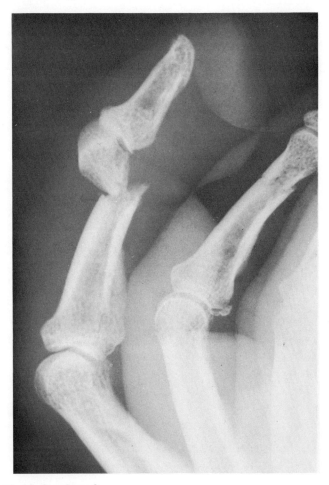

Figure 12–12. See Case 9.

DISCUSSION OF CASE 9.

The patient was admitted to the hospital and open reduction carried out. The distal fragment was brought down into proper alignment with the proximal fragment of the middle phalanx and pinned there with Kirschner wires. These were left in place four and a half weeks. Movement of the finger was started at the end of two weeks to diminish joint stiffness. He regained 40° flexion in the distal phalanx.

CASE 10—FINGER-RING INJURY

A fourteen-year-old boy had black devitalized tissue on the dorsum of his right ring finger (figure 12–13). Two weeks earlier, while jumping from a fence, he had caught his finger ring on the top of the fence. The ring tore the skin and subcutaneous tissue distally. (Distally based flaps have notoriously poor circulation.) He was treated primarily at another hospital, but the flap became infected. It is now infected and necrotic.

What should be done?

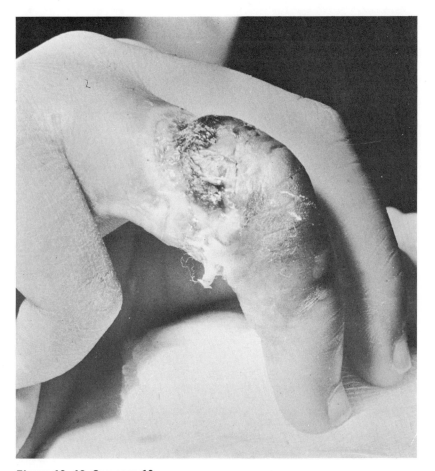

Figure 12–13. See case 10.

DISCUSSION OF CASE 10.

Procedure for injuries of this type should follow this order:

1. Culture the wound exudate.
2. Make gram stain of wound exudate.
3. Immediately start appropriate antibiotic (see chapter 11) while awaiting culture report on sensitivity.
4. Debride the dead tissue under anesthesia if no lymphangitis exists.
5. Apply local wet dressings such as 0.5% neomycin and change these q.i.d. (An alternate dressing would be one-half strength Dakin's solution.)
6. Carry out free skin graft when the wound is clean and healthy.

CASE 11—OPEN WOUND OF PALM WITH PROTRUDING MASS

A twelve-year-old boy is shown with a protruding mass at the ulnar border of the left hand (figure 12—14). He had fallen on broken glass one month earlier. His mother noted this mass two weeks after injury. The mass appeared to be covered with granulation tissue and pulsated questionably. There was a bruit on auscultation over the hypothenar eminence.

How should this protruding mass be treated?

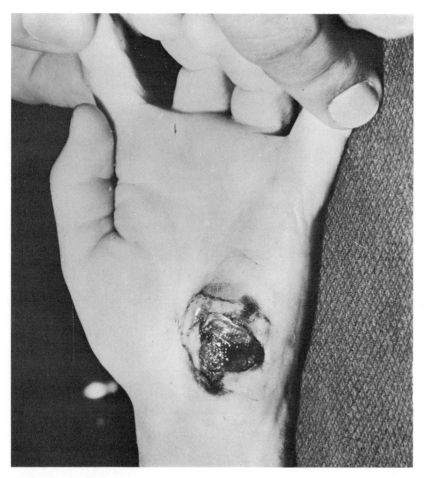

Figure 12—14. See case 11.

DISCUSSION OF CASE 11.

At operation, the ulnar artery was identified proximal to the mass. Control was obtained with a small rubber drain. The mass was then opened and found to be a false aneurysm. At the base were two lumina of the ulnar artery. One side of the artery had been cut away, leaving the proximal and distal lumina open but separated. The adjacent ulnar nerve was intact. The artery was reanastomosed under magnification. The ulnar pulse remained good. The wound healed satisfactorily, and the patient regained normal use of his hand.

CASE 12—HEMOPHILIA WITH SWOLLEN PALM

A nine-year-old boy with known hemophilia played basketball the day before admission and developed acute swelling of his right palm and thenar eminence (figure 12–15).

What is the diagnosis and treatment?

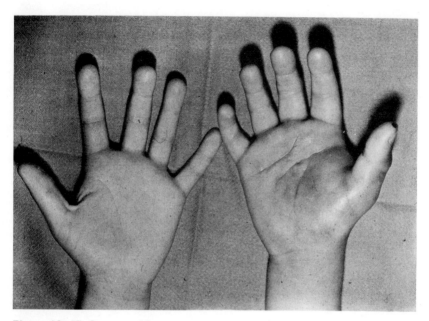

Figure 12–15. See case 12.

DISCUSSION OF CASE 12.

The swelling is the result of hemorrhage into palmar and thenar tissues. (He had no fever, and there was no wound of entrance to indicate an infection.)

Elevation, gentle compression of the palmar tissues, and continued observation of the circulation of the fingertips were carried out.

Whole blood transfusions were given. Cryoprecipitated factor VIII would be used now.

CASE 13—PAINFUL FINGERTIP

Redness and swelling of the tip of the left ring finger (figure 12–16) of a fifteen-year-old boy started along the radial border of the finger three days earlier. Penicillin had been given and a small incision made on the finger two days before, but the process had become worse, producing throbbing pain.

What is the diagnosis, and what treatment is indicated?

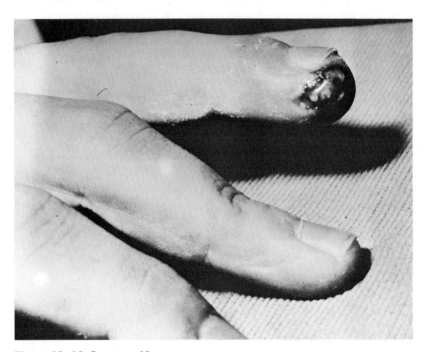

Figure 12–16. See case 13.

DISCUSSION OF CASE 13.

The present condition of the finger, despite previous treatment, indicates distal closed-space infection of the left ring finger (felon).

The boy was admitted to the hospital. Wide incision and drainage along the radial border of the tip of the finger, dividing the ligaments between periosteum and skin, was carried out. One-half milliliter of thick pus was released. The wound was held open with vaseline wick. Cultures were made, and heavy doses of erythromycin (500 mgm q.i.d.) were administered. The next day the culture showed staphylococcus that was resistant to penicillin but sensitive to erythromycin, which was continued. The infection cleared, and the wound healed spontaneously (see also chapter 11).

CASE 14—ROLLER INJURY

A seventy-five-year-old woman caught her left hand in the rollers of a clothes wringer thirteen days before figure 12–17 was taken. The skin is necrotic over the extensor tendon and the M-P joint of the index finger.

What procedure is indicated?

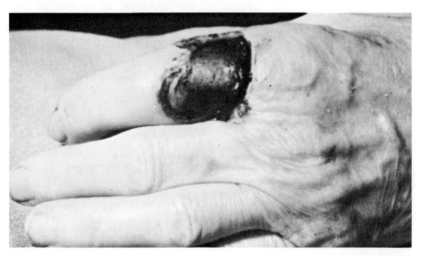

Figure 12–17. See Case 14.

DISCUSSION OF CASE 14.

In order to save the joint and the extensor tendon, a local flap of skin was shifted distally from the dorsum of the hand after excision of the necrotic tissues, exposing the tendon and the joint. A free skin graft was utilized to close the defect created by the shifted flap and to close that part of the wound where the tendon was not exposed. The result four and a half years later is shown in figure 12–18.

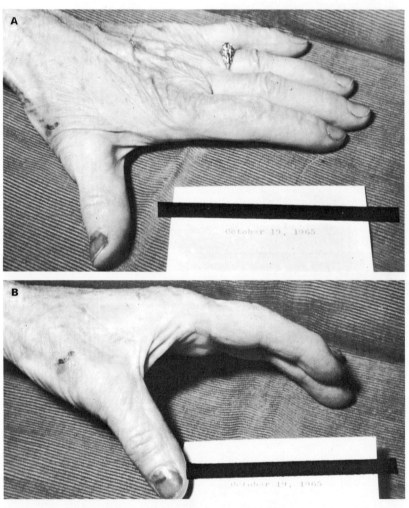

Figure 12–18. The result of the repair of the left hand of the patient in figure 12–17, four and a half years later. The shifted skin flaps and free skin graft are well healed. The finger moves with very little restriction.

CASE 15—COMPOUND INJURY

This twenty-nine-year-old man's left hand was caught in an industrial rubber mixer shortly before figure 12–19 was made. The fingers and thumb are severely mangled and partially amputated, and the skin avulsed. The entire dorsal skin of the hand is also avulsed.

How should treatment proceed?

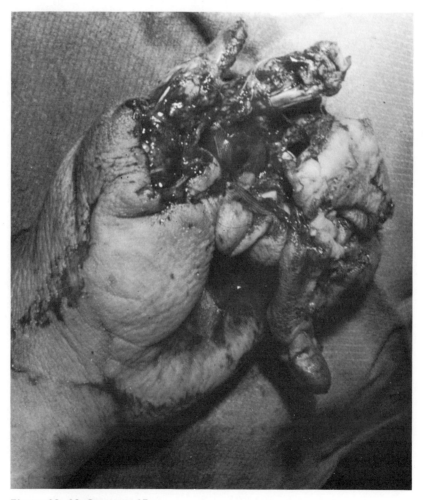

Figure 12–19. See case 15.

DISCUSSION OF CASE 15.

There are so many things wrong in this injury that it is hard to know where to start. In a severe case, such as this, the following is a good plan:

1. Cleanse the wound extensively to diminish the hazard of infection. The surrounding skin should be shaved and scrubbed with detergent and the fingernails cleaned and cut short. This should be followed by copious irrigation of the wound with normal saline solution. The whole process should then be repeated with a second new setup.
2. Trim away devitalized tissues sparingly.
3. Regain skeletal alignment as much as possible using internal fixation.
5. Gain closure by suture and skin graft unless contamination is severe or the case is seen late after injury.

This outline is essentially the method used for the hand injury in figure 12–19. Some additional skin was lost, and regrafting of skin was carried out on three subsequent occasions. The cleft between the thumb and index finger was deepened with a Z-plasty. The final result is shown in figure 12–20.

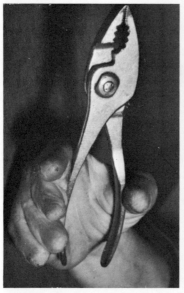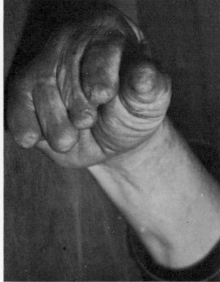

Figure 12–20. See case 15.

INDEX